# SURGERY & MEDICINE

## AN IMAGE ARCHIVE FOR
## ARTISTS *And* DESIGNERS

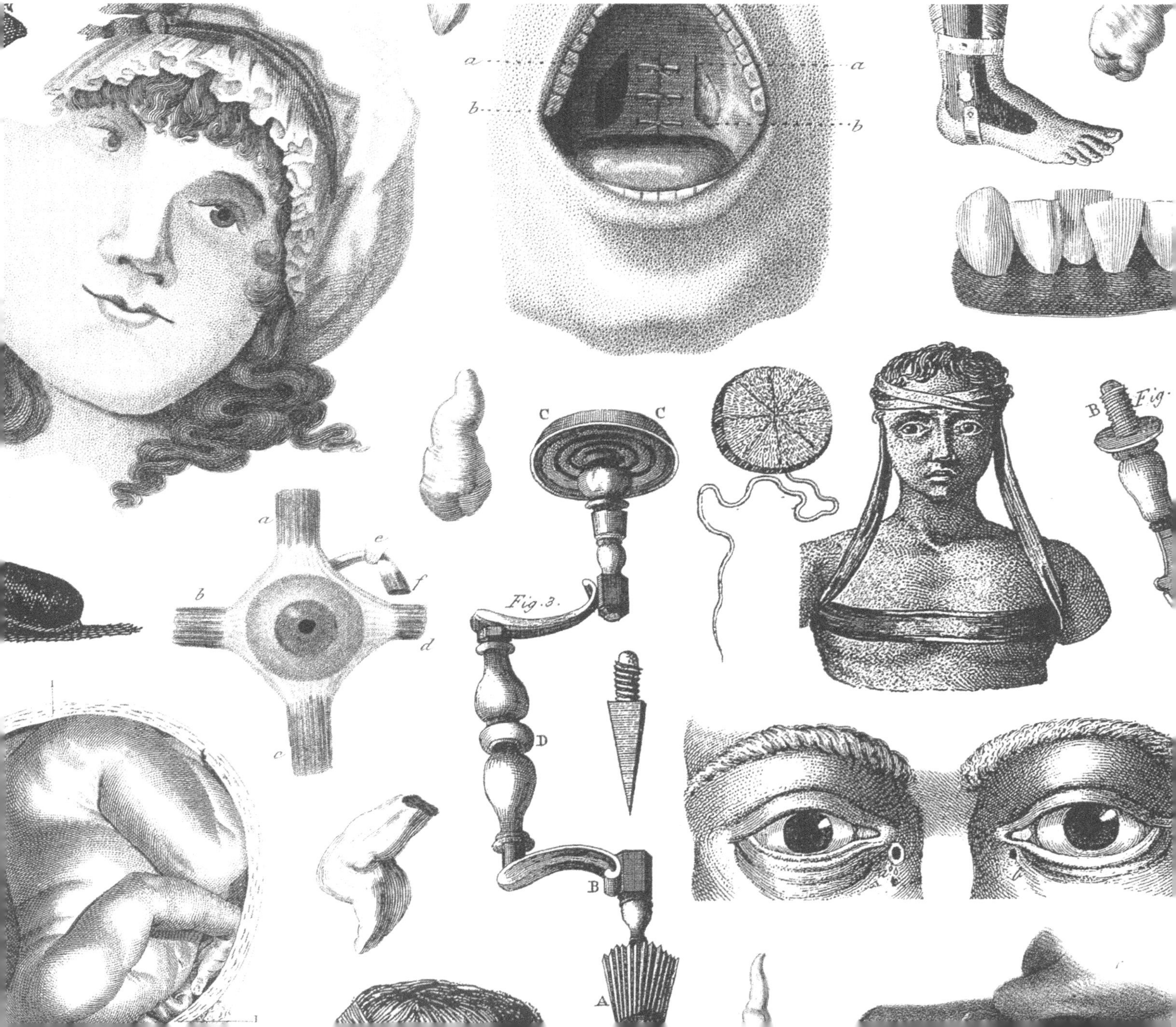

# INTRODUCTION

SURGERY AND MEDICINE

Are you looking to gain access to hundreds of beautifully rendered vintage medial and surgical illustrations to use in graphic design projects, collages and fine art projects? Alternatively, are you looking for the best reference material available for your own vintage medical inspired illustrations and designs?

*Surgery and Medicine: An Image Archive of Vintage Medical Images for Artists and Designers* will provide you with precisely that. This book is a brilliantly curated resource that will provide you with precisely that. This book features a fascinating curated collection of 17th and 18th-century engravings, etchings and lithographs exploring dentistry, eye surgery, amputation, rhinoplasty, prosthetics, bandages and dressing, childbirth, surgical tools and much more.

We hope you enjoy this resource.

*Copyright*
Copyright ©Avenue House Press Pty Ltd 2020.

*Bibliographical Note*
This book is a new work created by Avenue House Press Pty Ltd.

ISBN: 978-1-925968-38-5

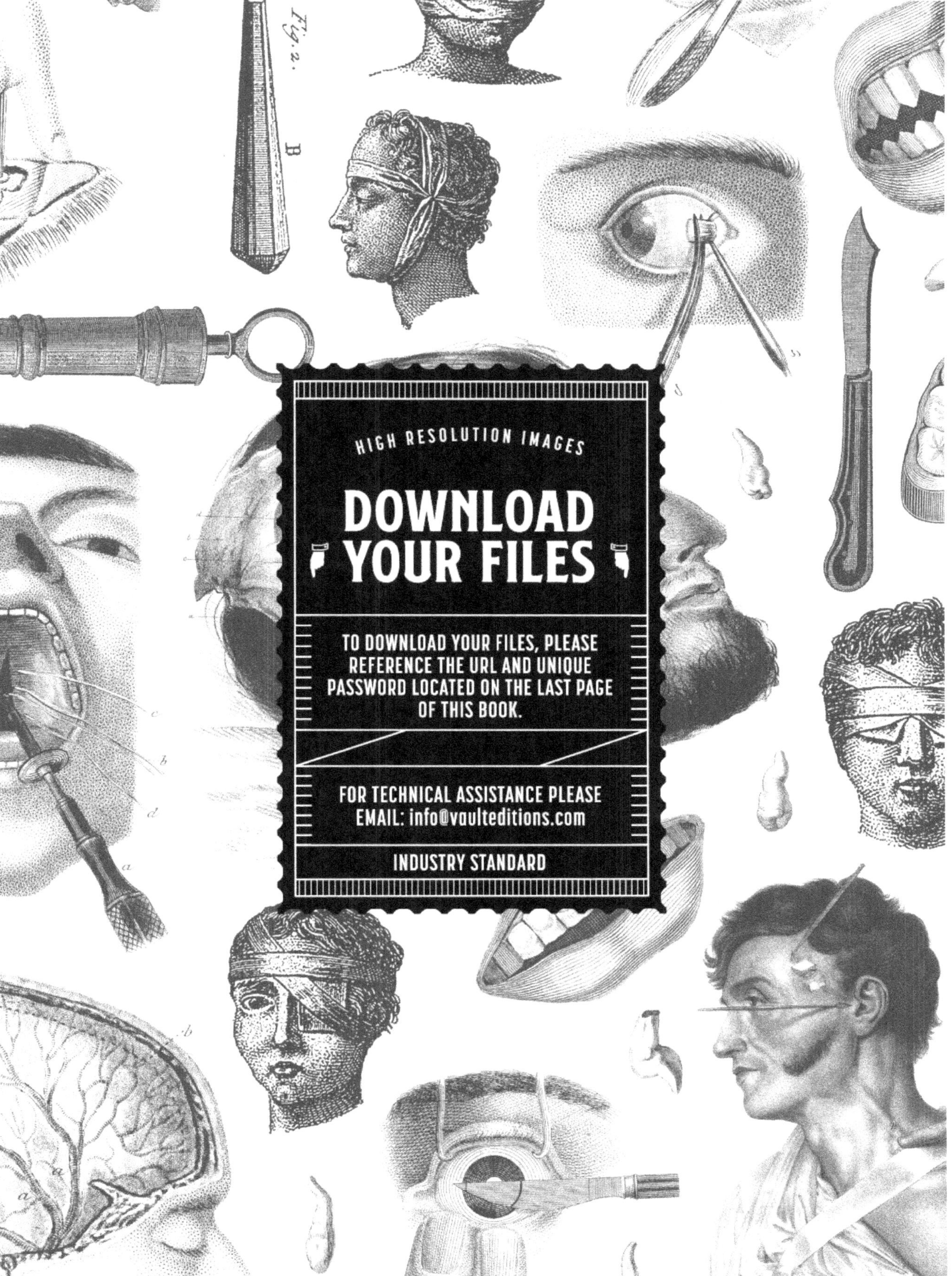
HIGH RESOLUTION IMAGES
DOWNLOAD YOUR FILES
TO DOWNLOAD YOUR FILES, PLEASE REFERENCE THE URL AND UNIQUE PASSWORD LOCATED ON THE LAST PAGE OF THIS BOOK.
FOR TECHNICAL ASSISTANCE PLEASE EMAIL: info@vaulteditions.com
INDUSTRY STANDARD

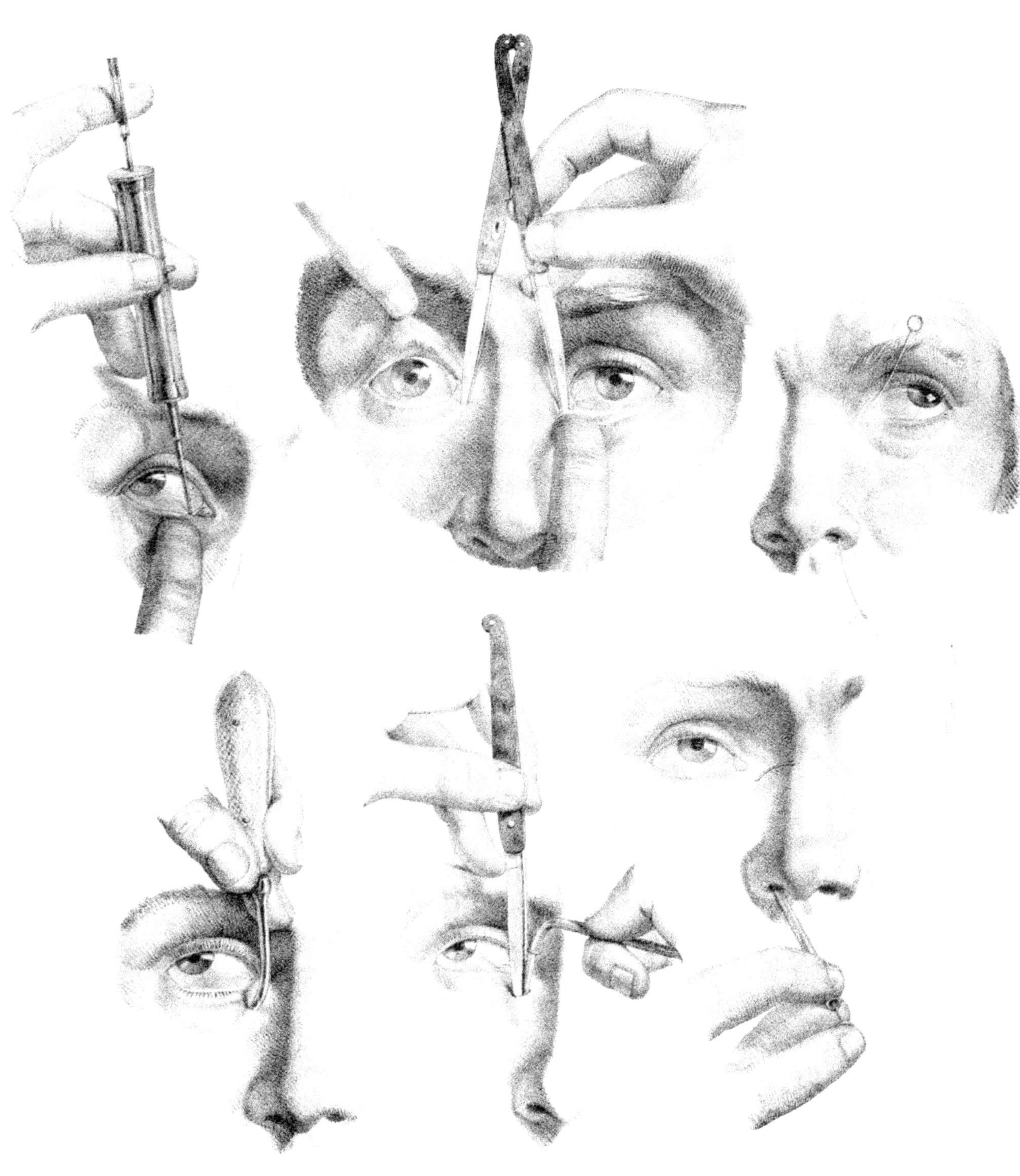

01: Surgery on the lacrimal glands and ducts.

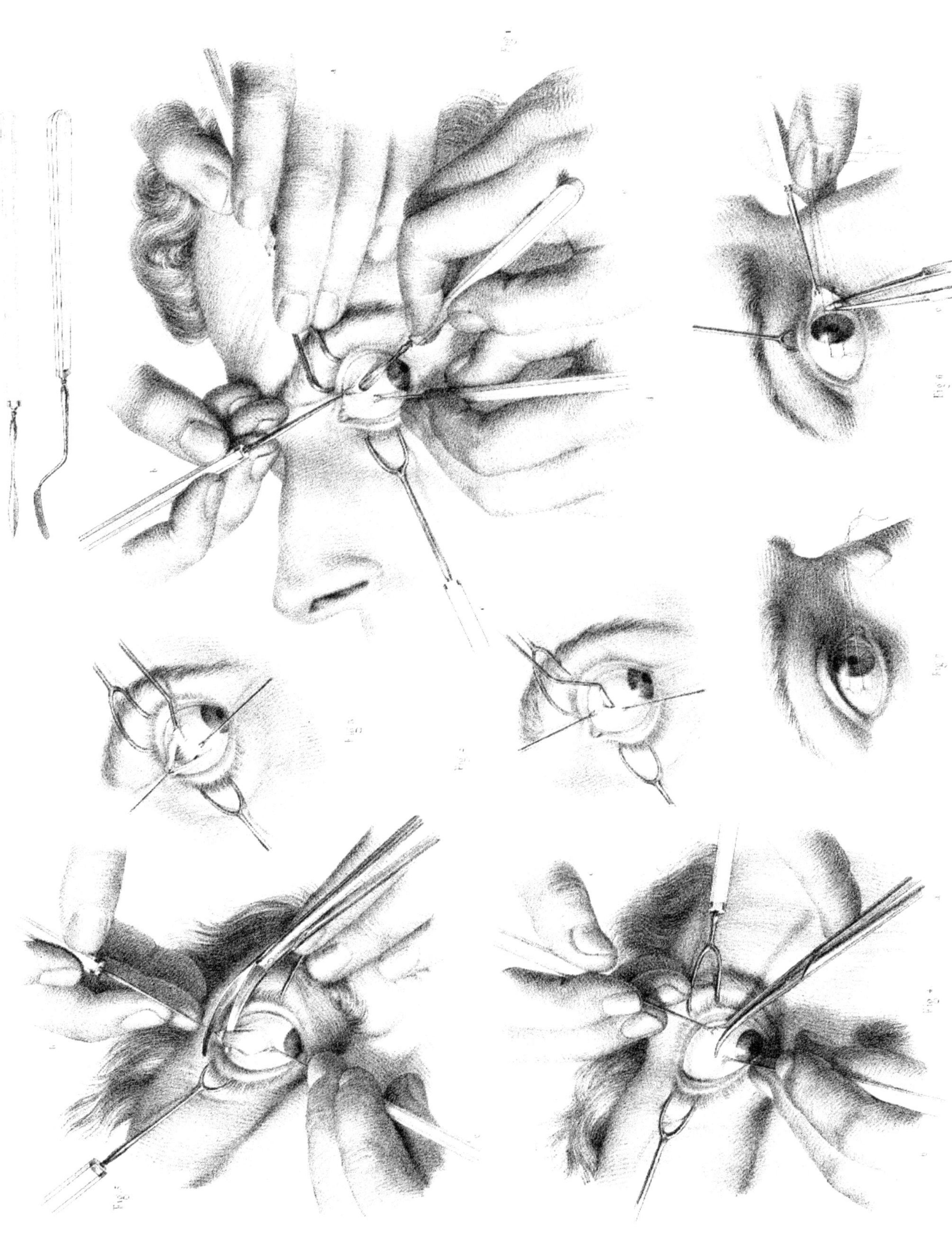

03

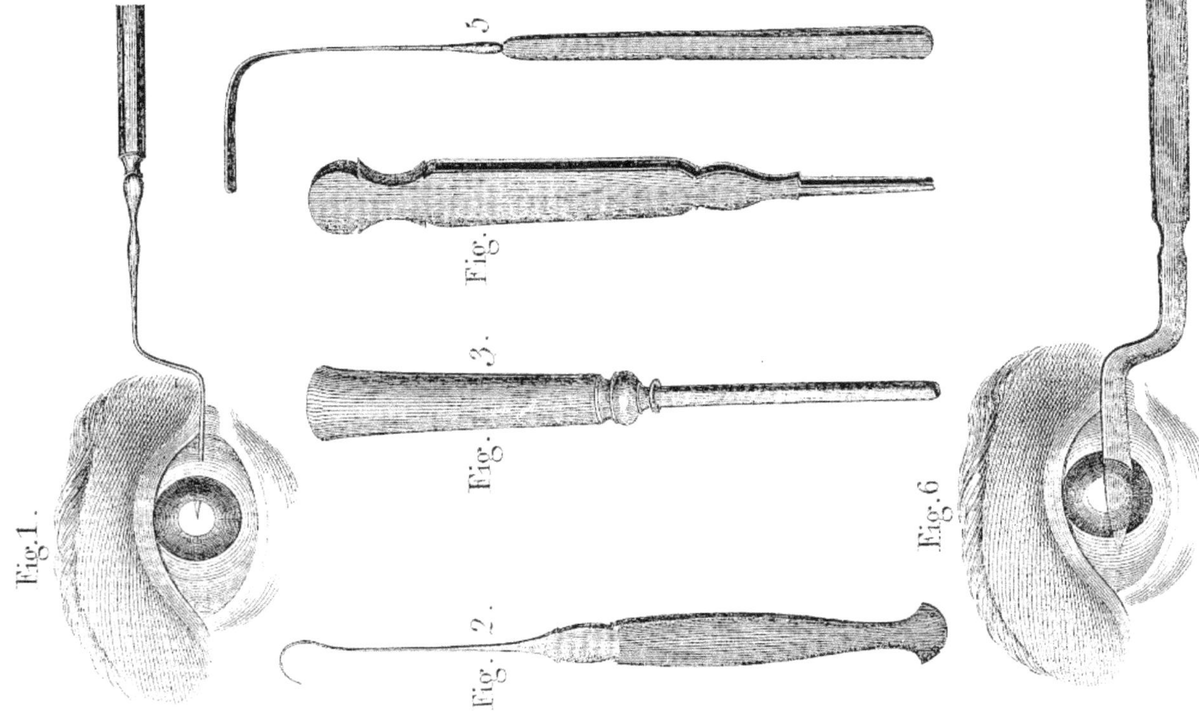



04

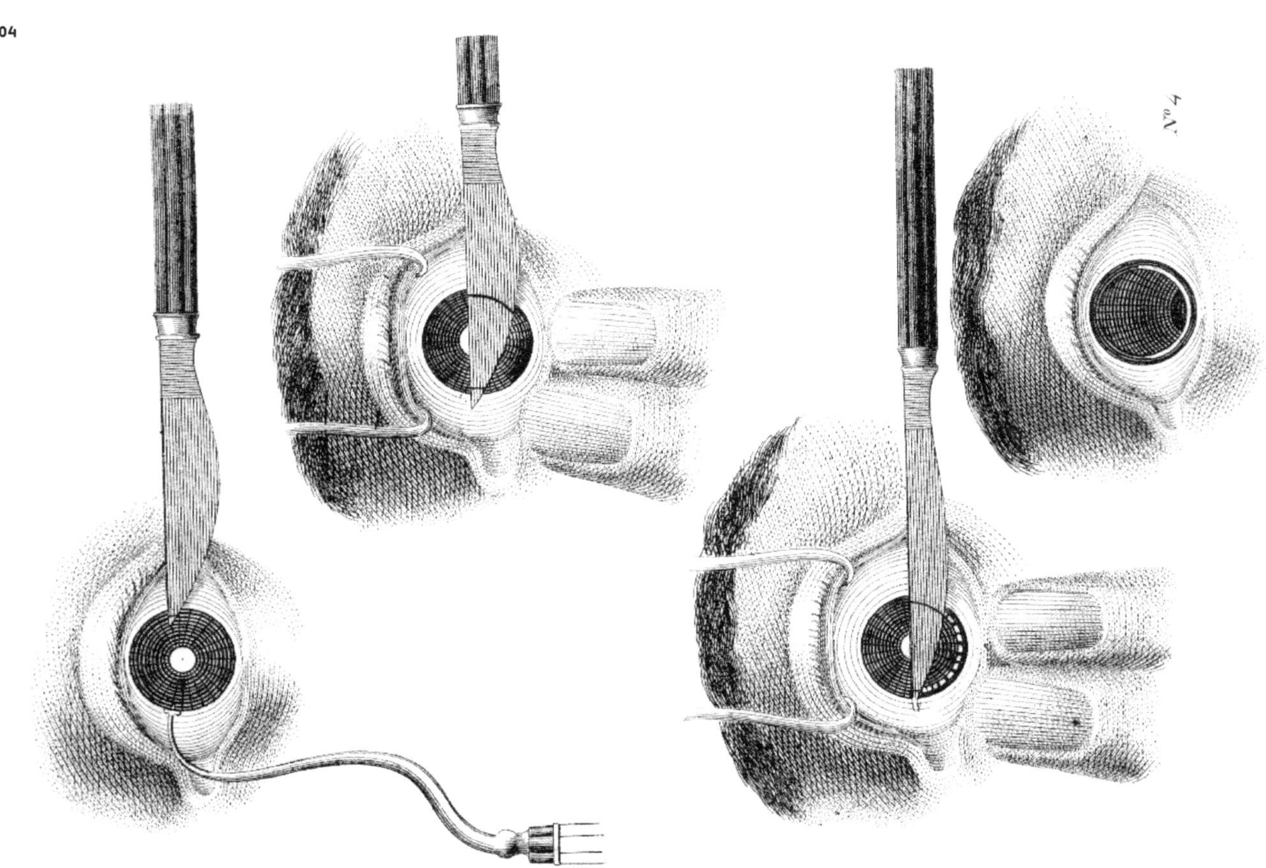

03: Eye surgery to remove cataracts.          04: Eye surgery to remove cataracts.

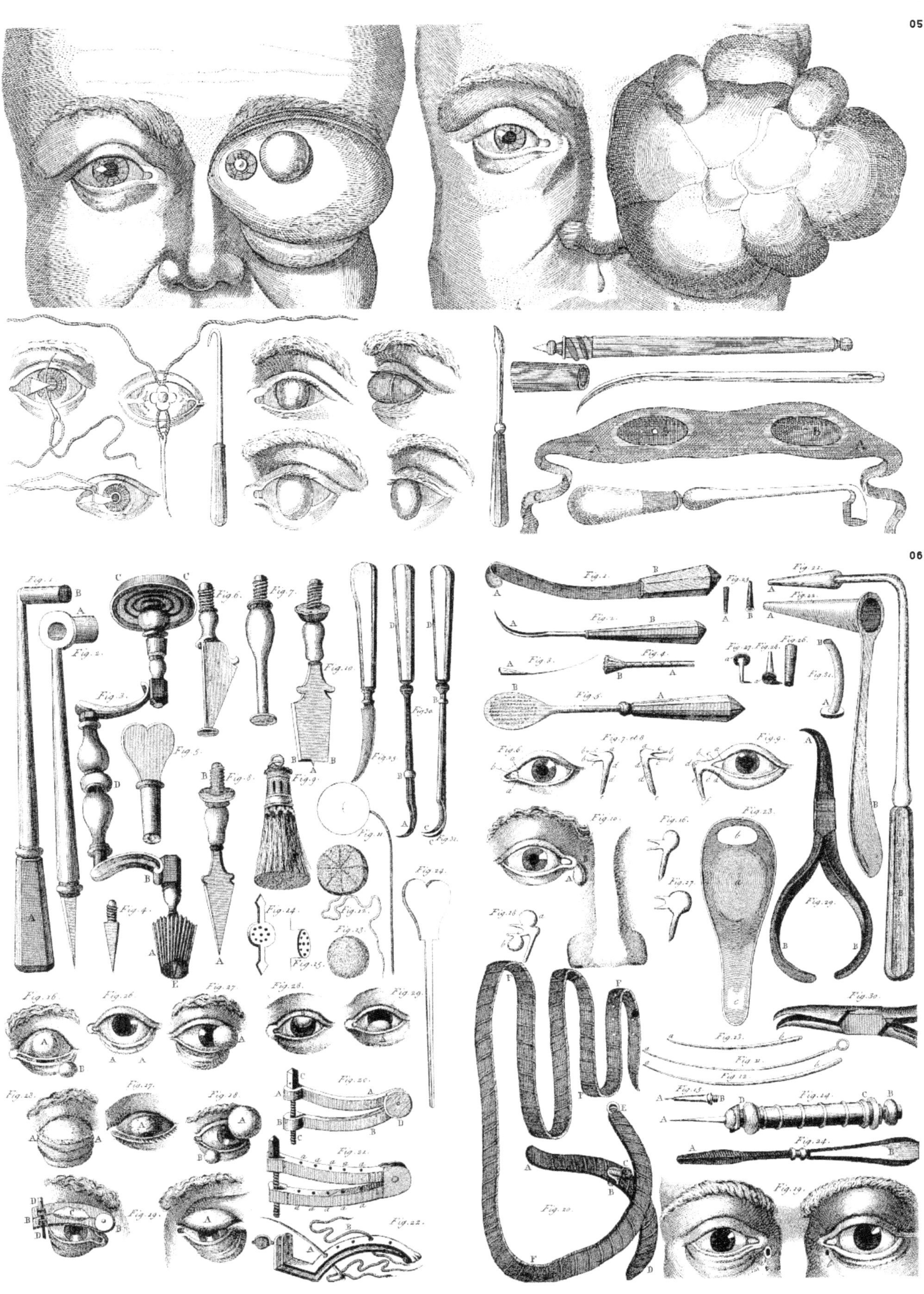



SURGERY AND MEDICINE

05: Eye diseases and surgical instruments.      06: Surgical instruments.

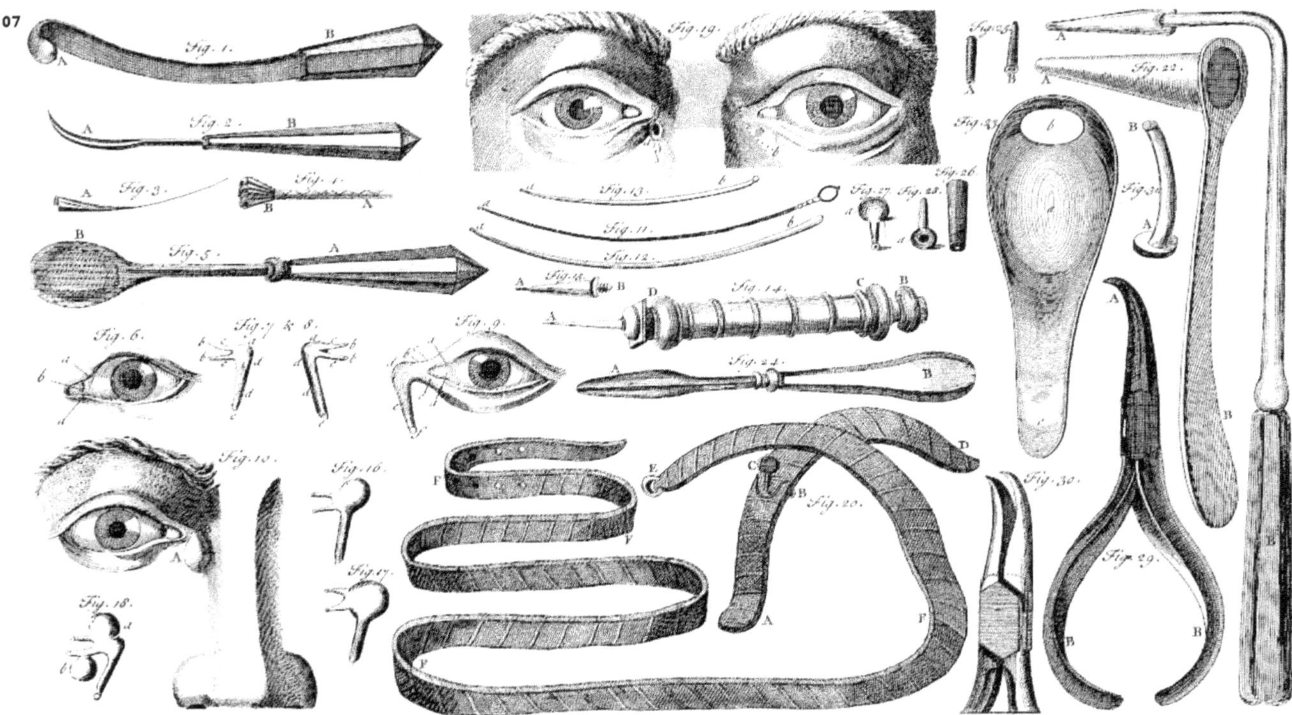

07

08

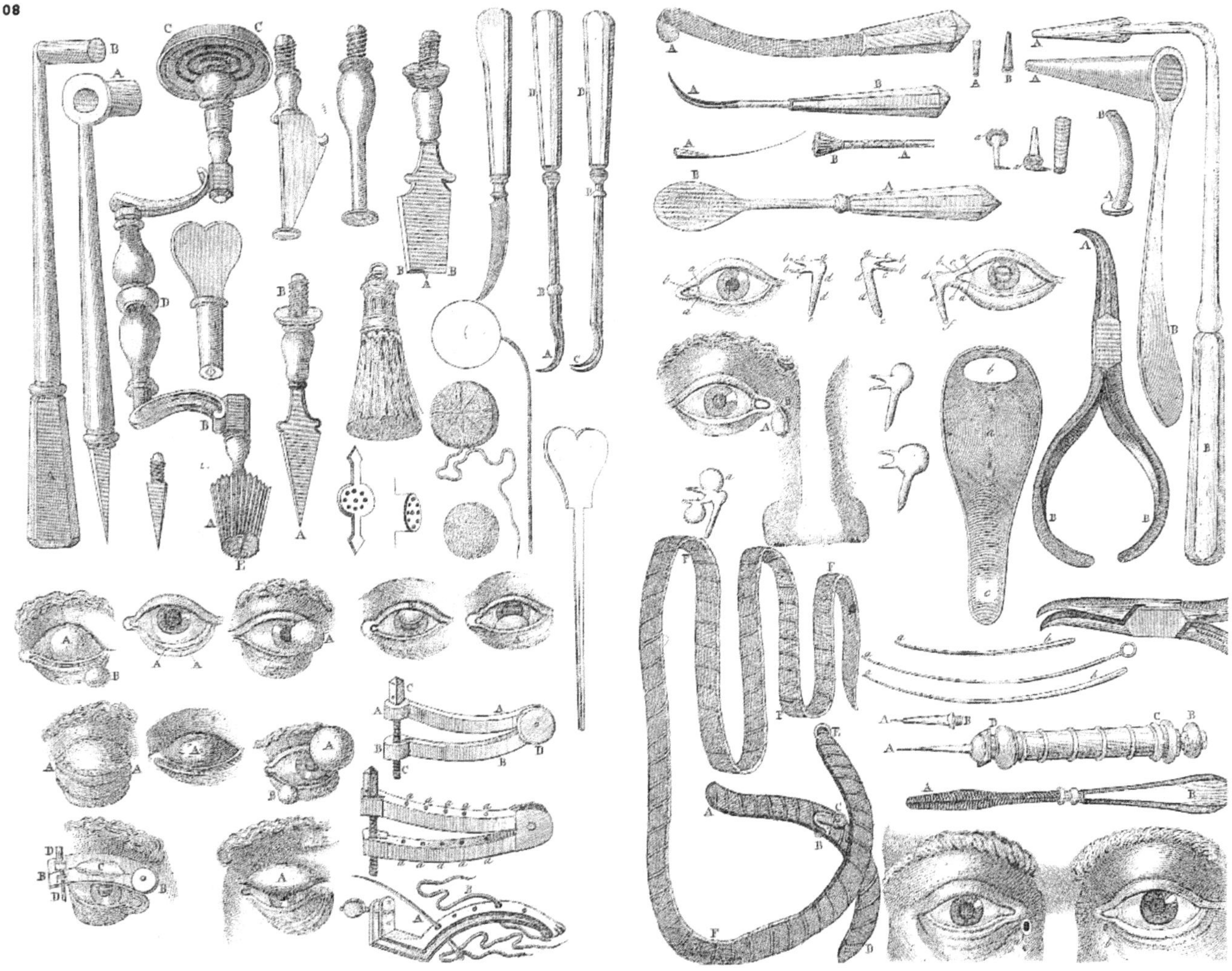

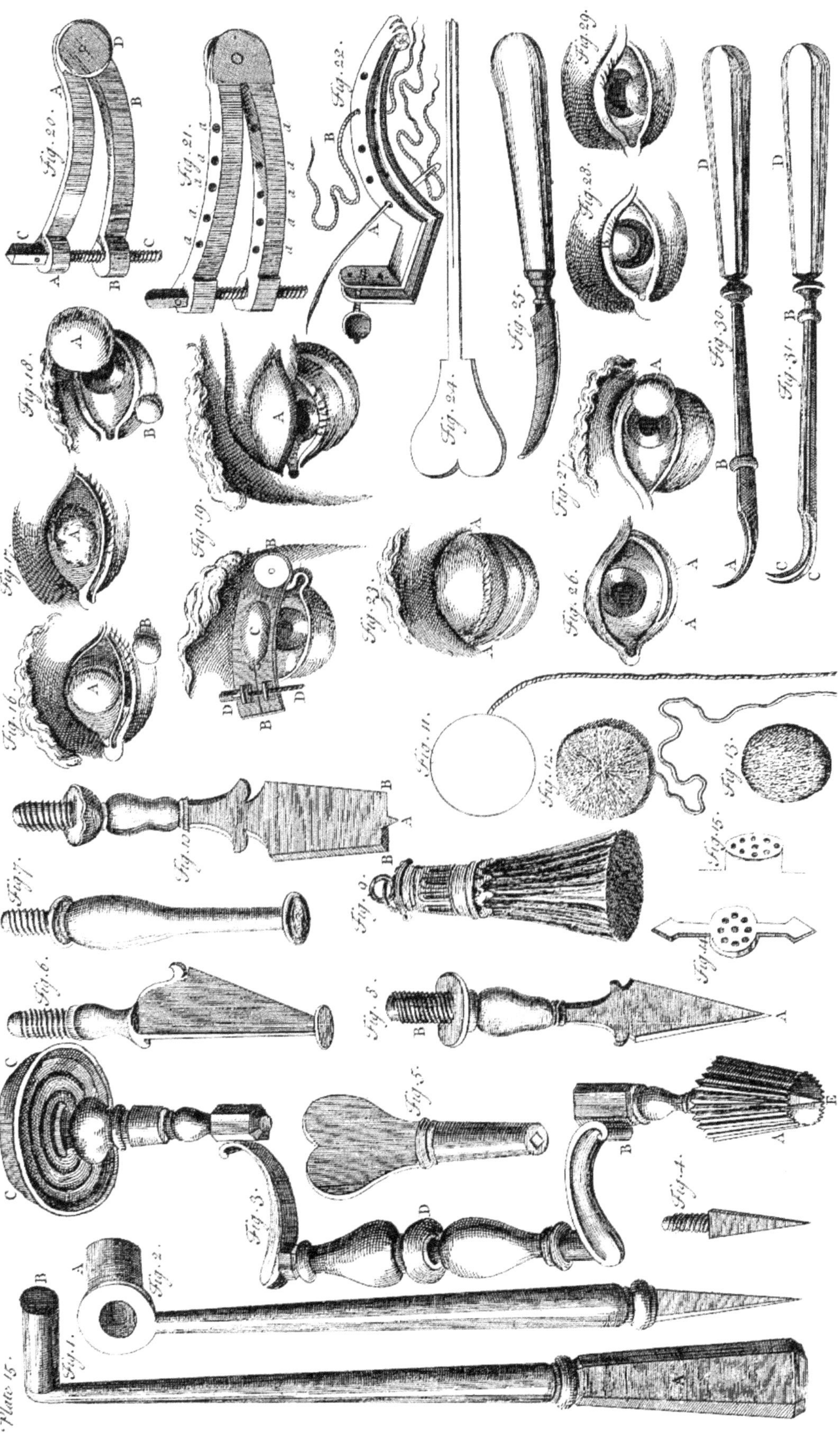



09: Surgical Instruments.

10



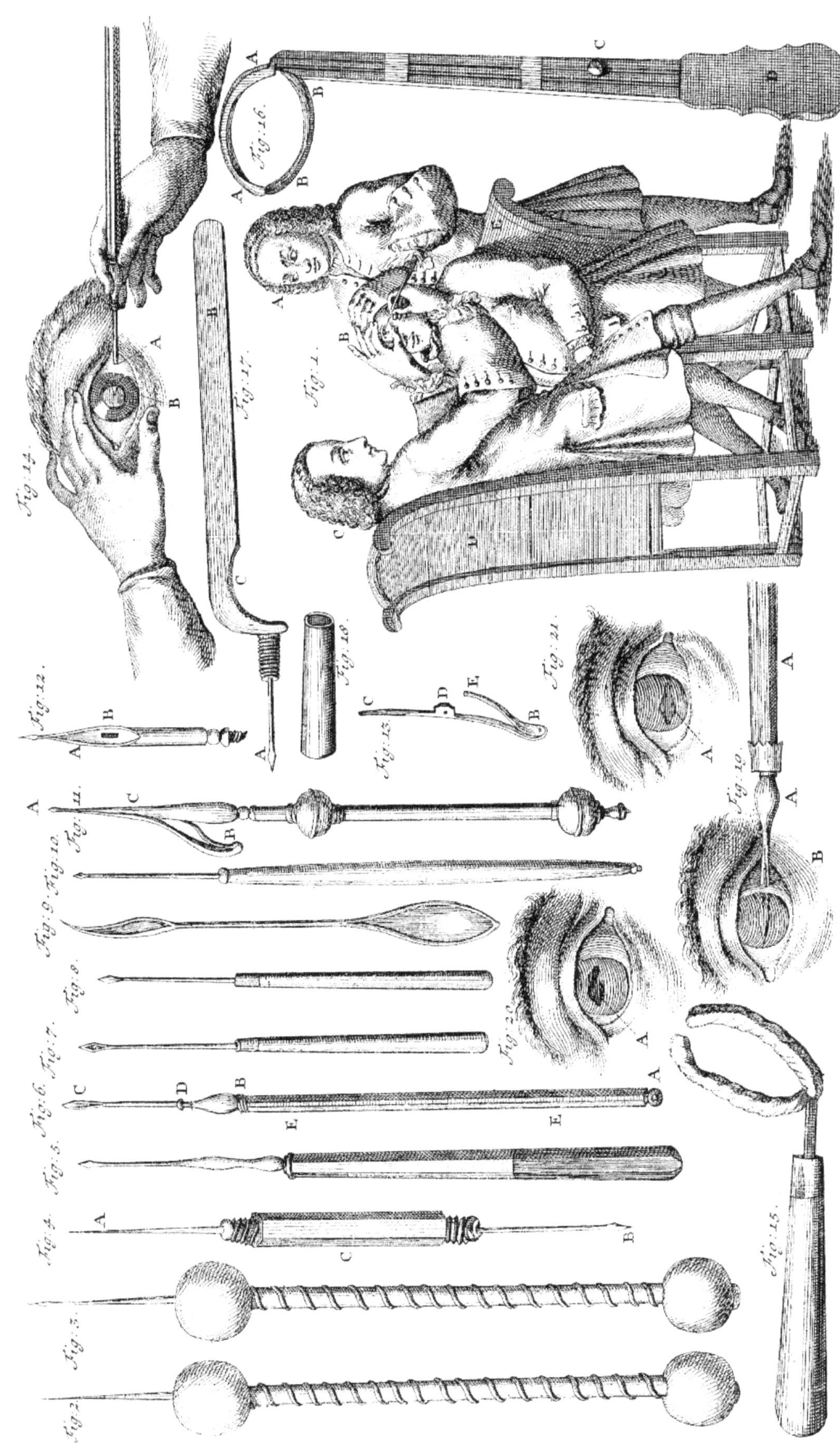

10: Surgical instruments and patients
undergoing treatment.

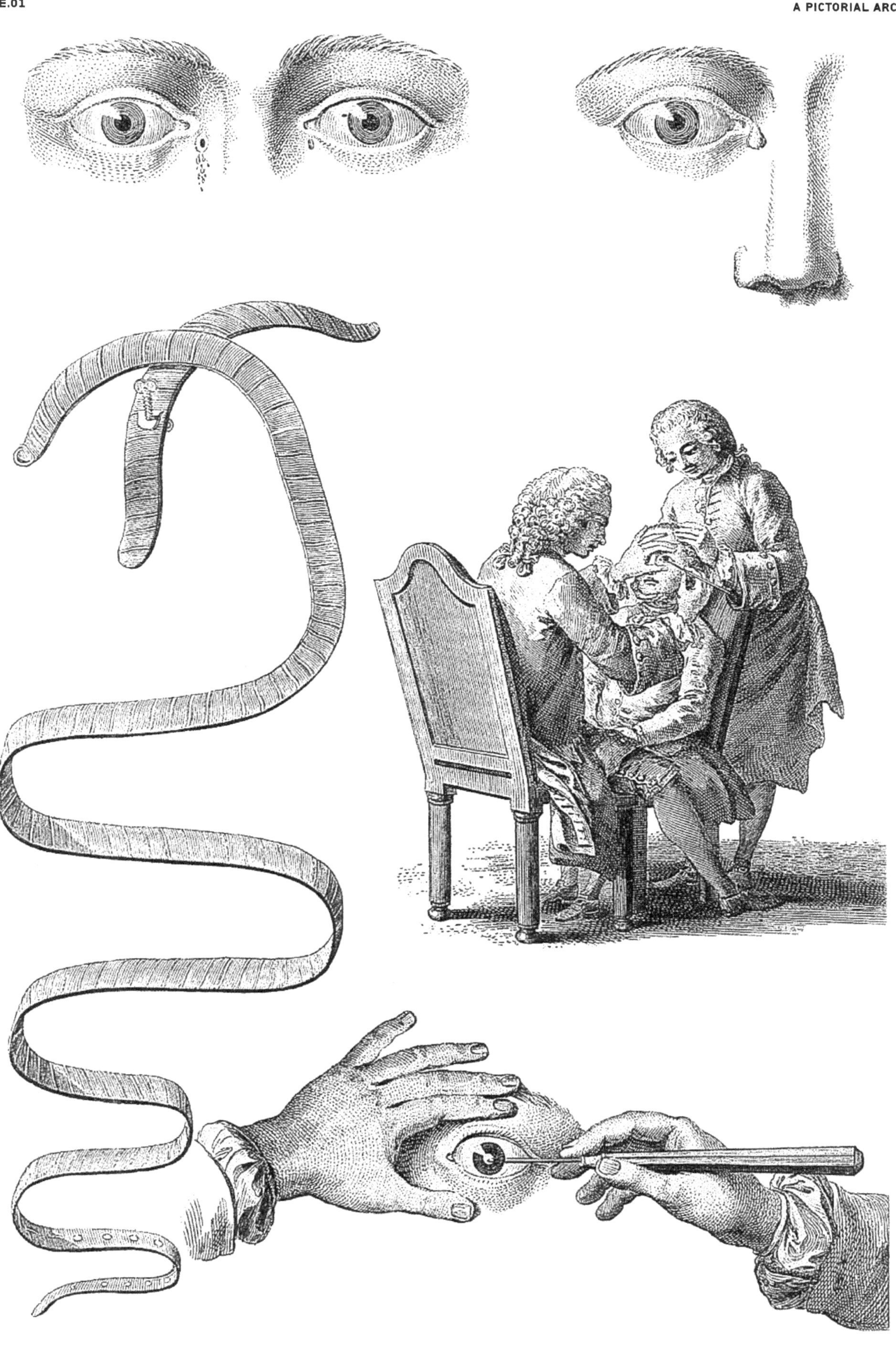



11: instruments for the treatment of cataracts
and fistulas of the lacrimal canals.

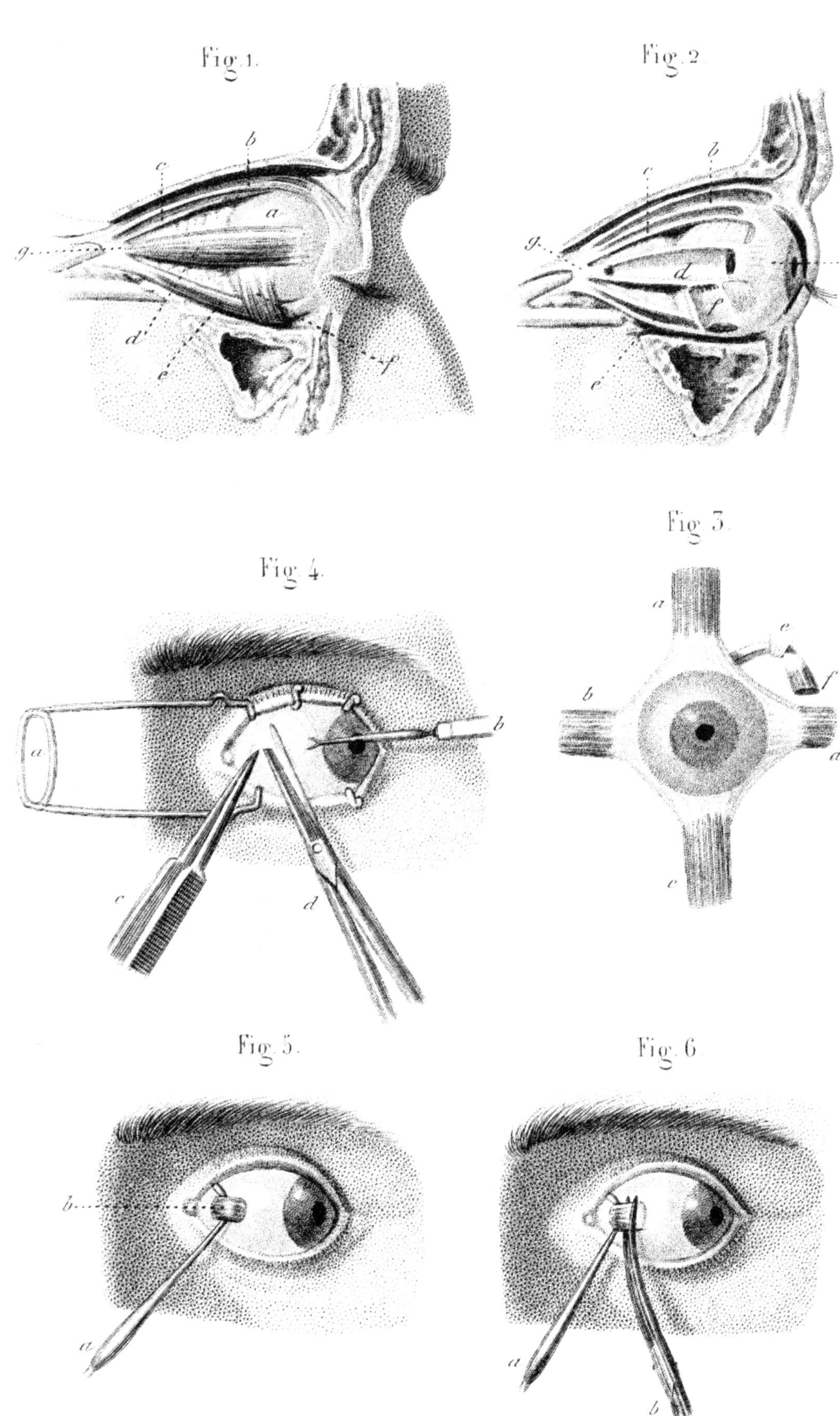


12: Illustration of surgery on the eye.

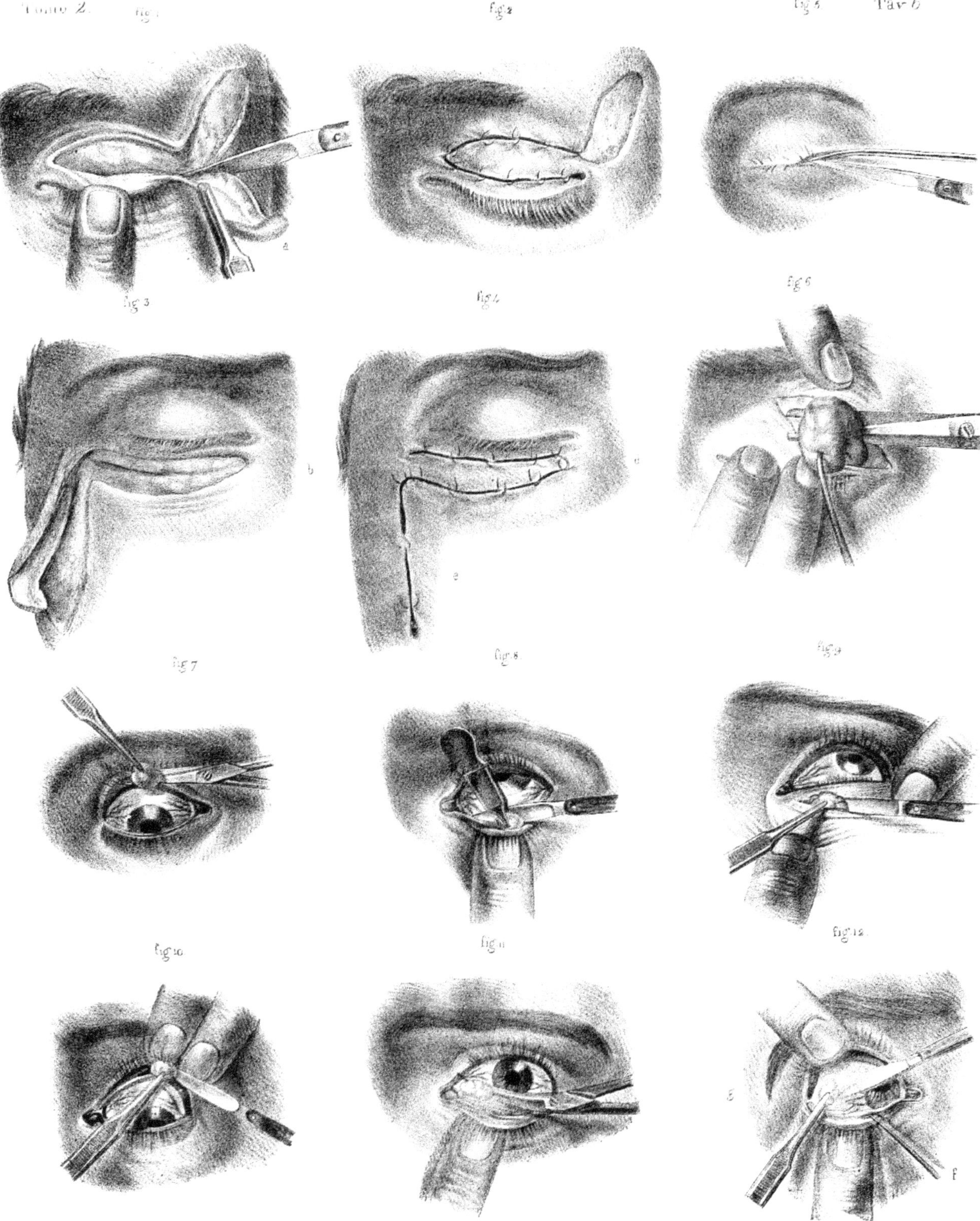

13: Method of surgery practiced on the eyelids.

14



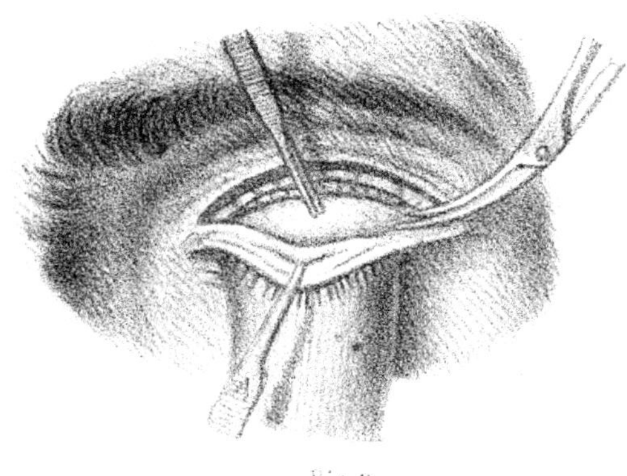

Fig. 2.

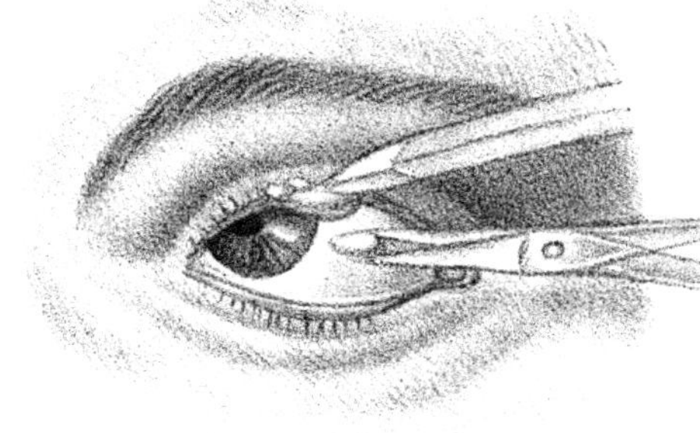

Fig. 1.

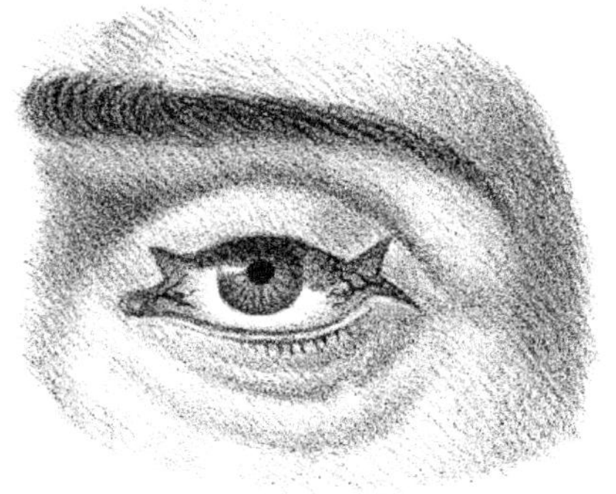

Fig. 4.

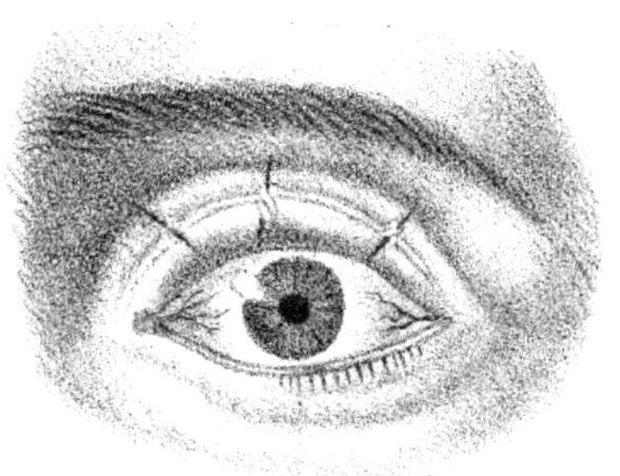

Fig. 3.

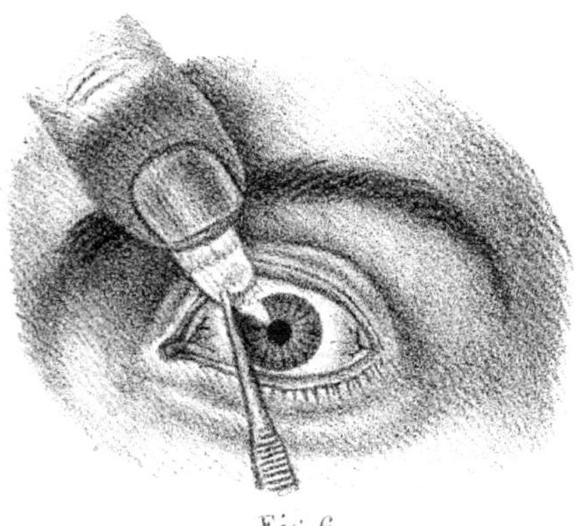

Fig. 6.

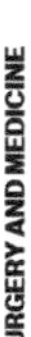

Fig. 5.

14: Method of surgery practiced on the eyelids.

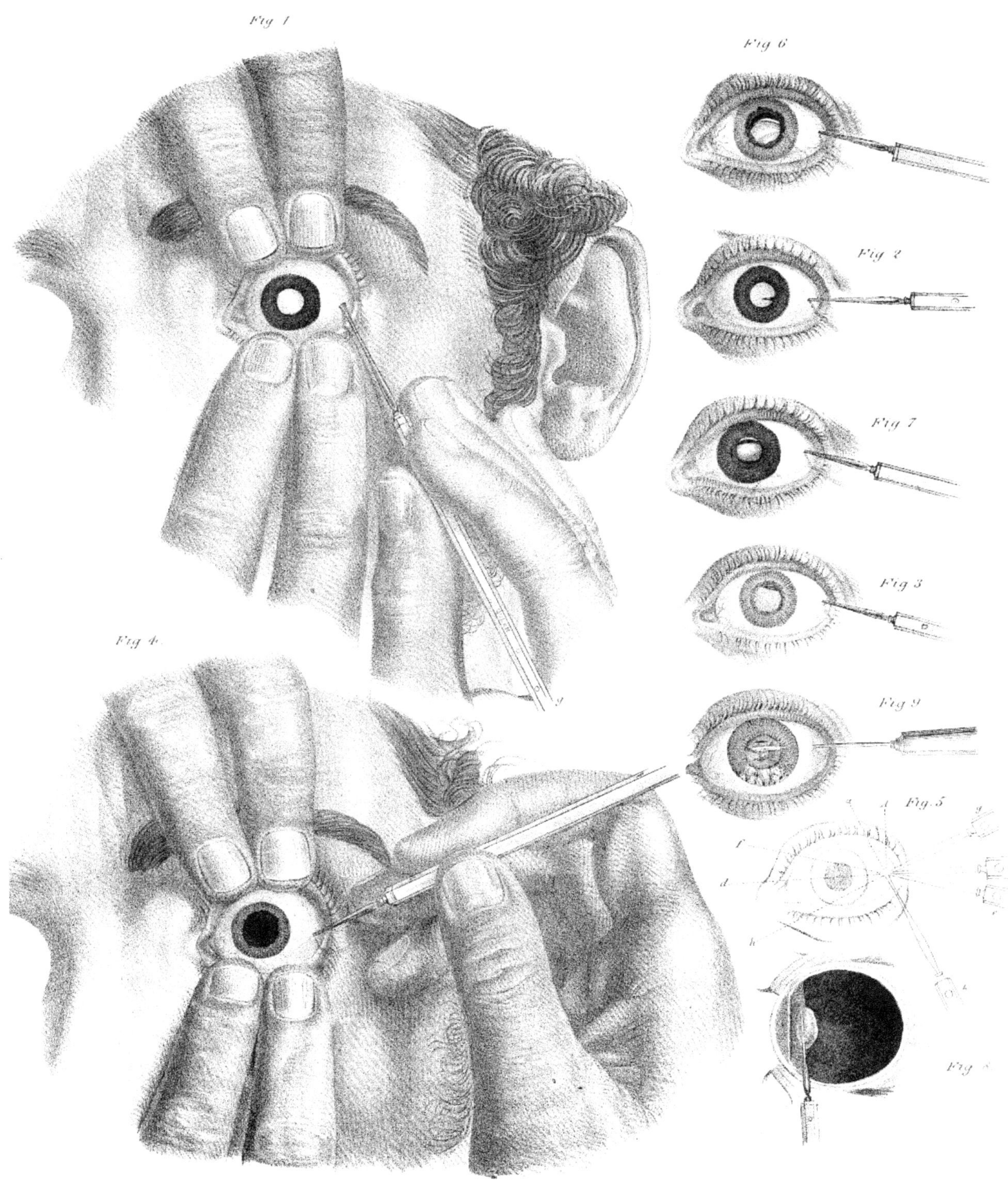




15: Illustration of surgery on the eye for the
removal of a cataract.

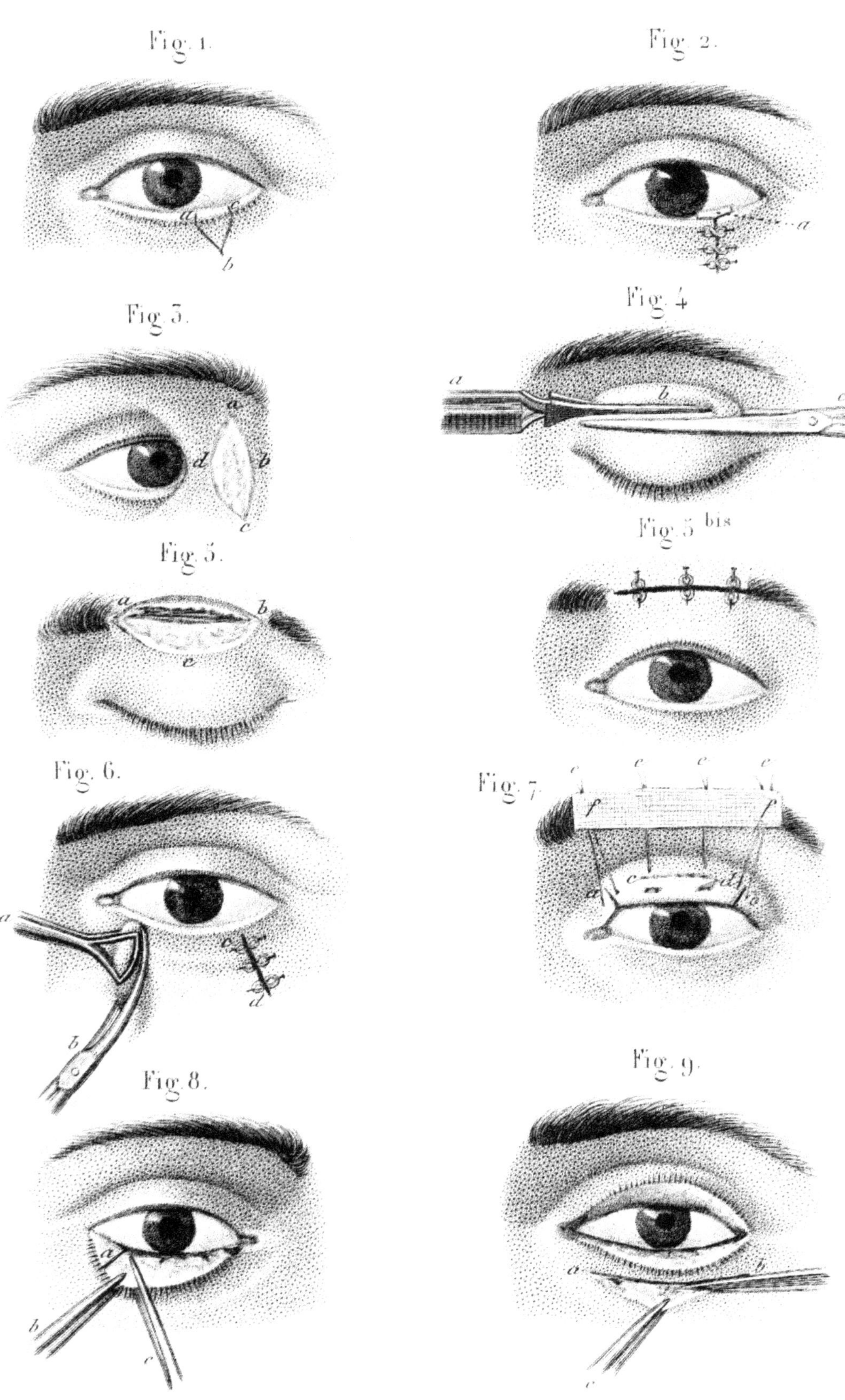


16: Surgery on the upper and lower eyelids.

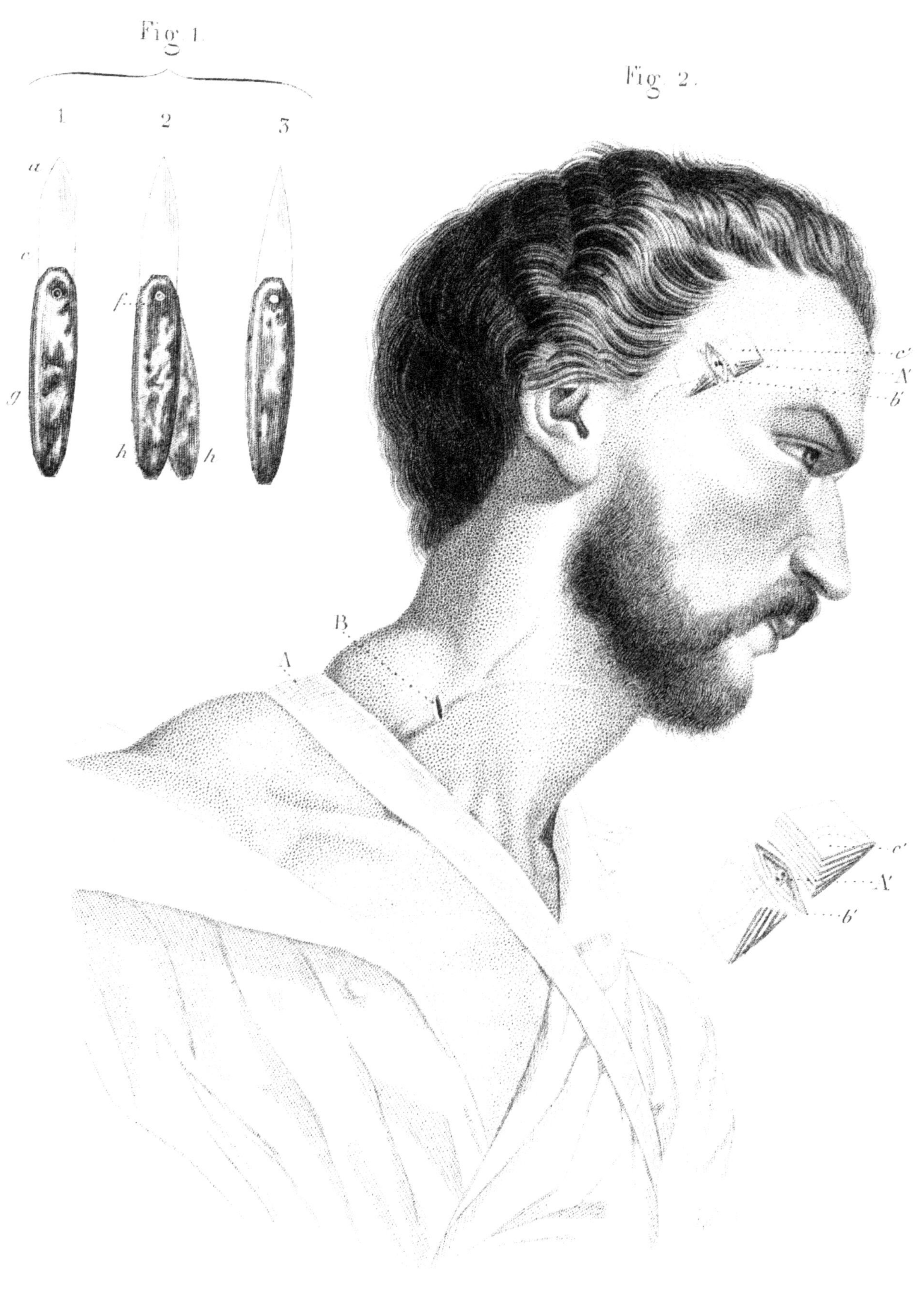




17: Illustration of lancets and incision points.

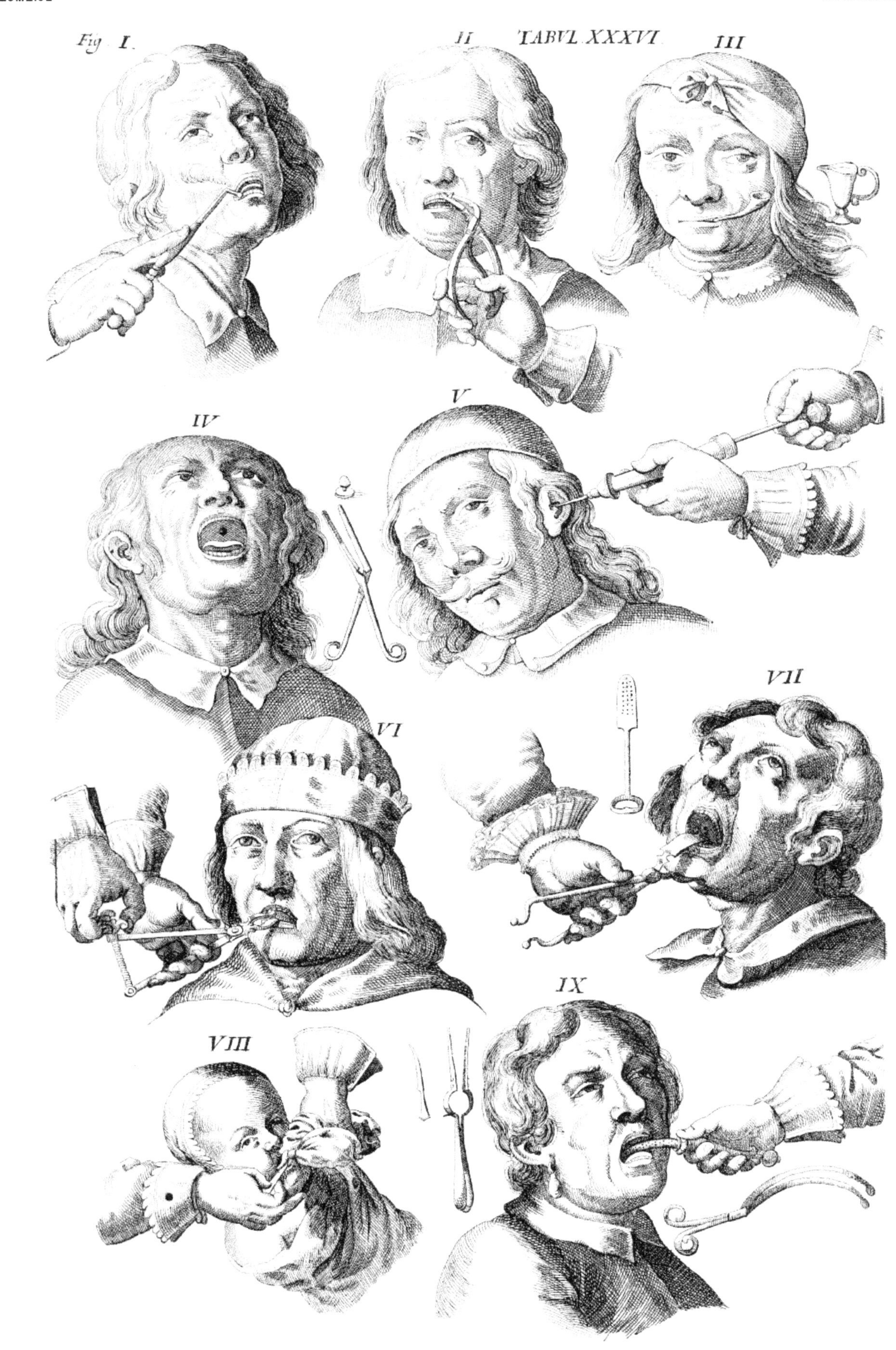


18: Mouth and ear surgical procedures.

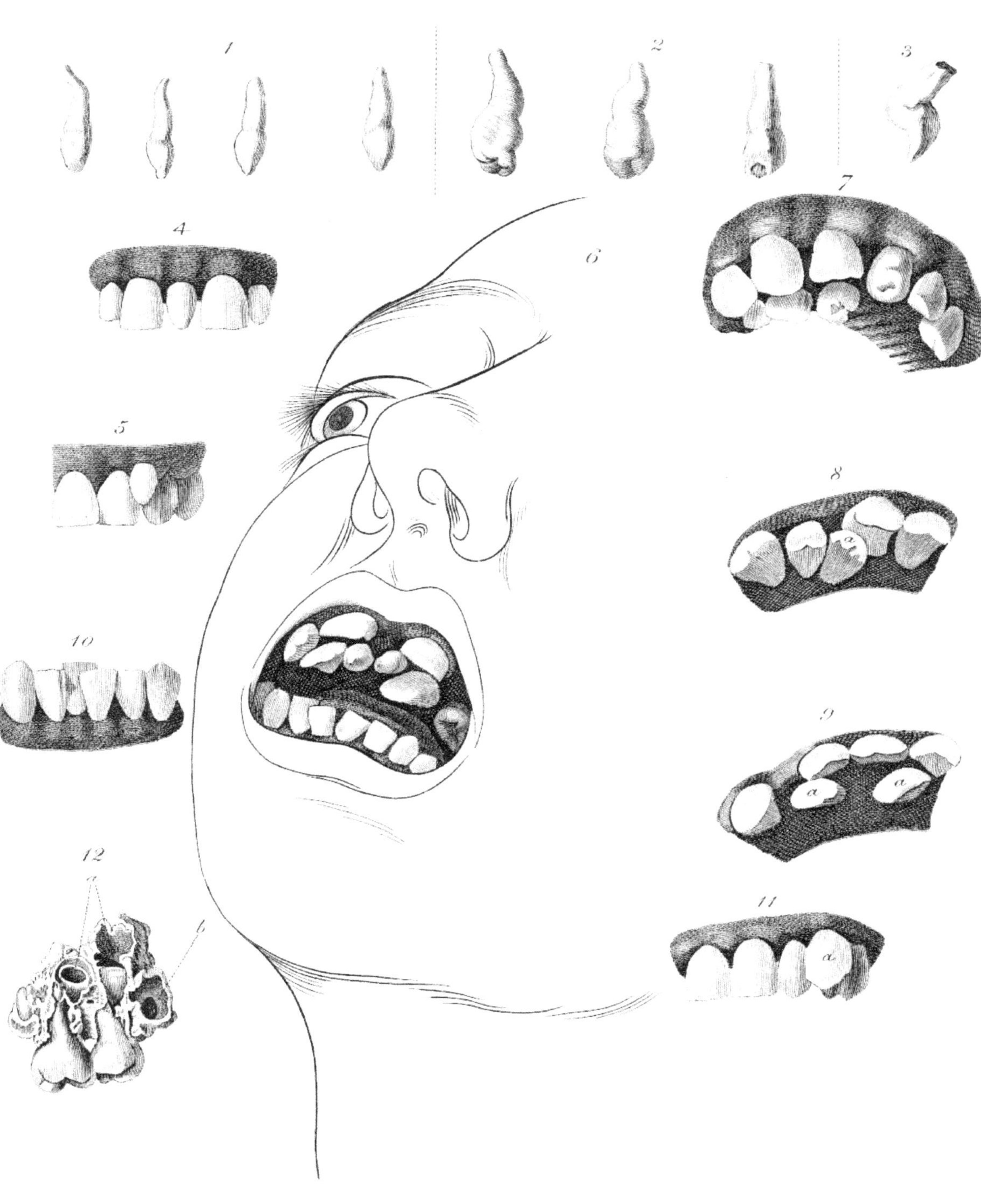



19: Cases of supernumerary teeth.

20

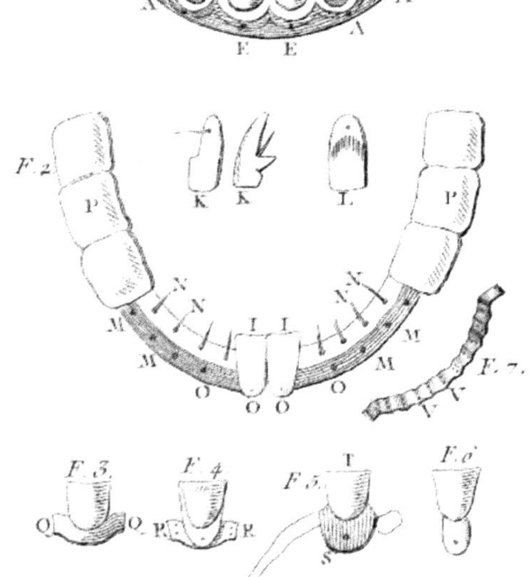

22

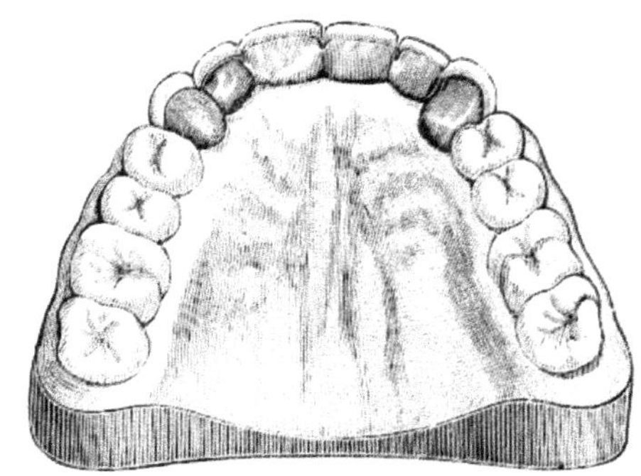

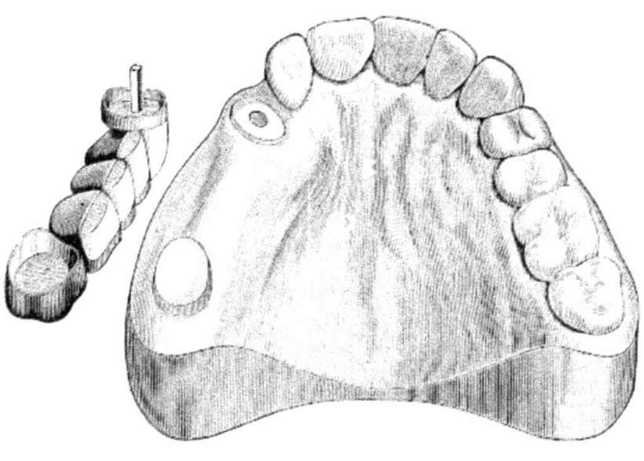

21

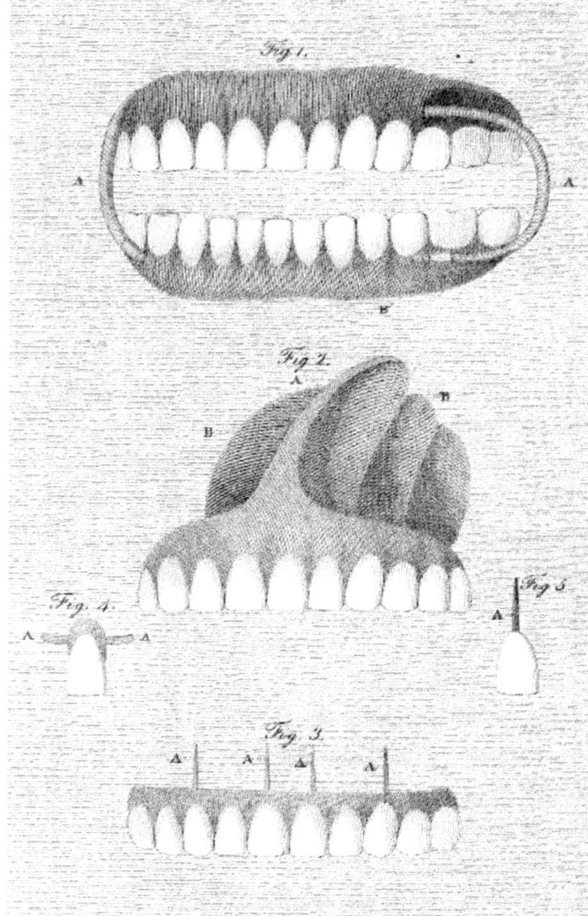

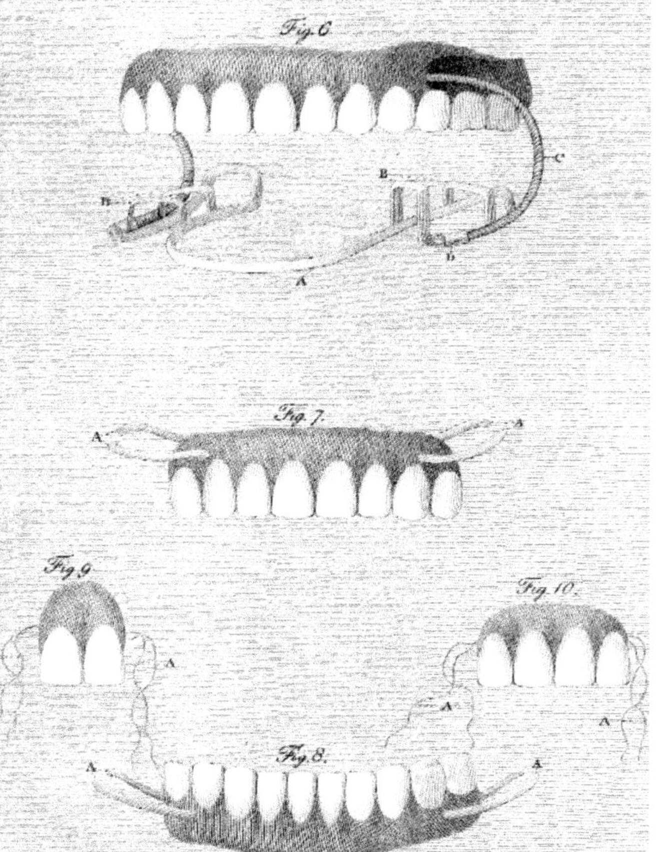

20: Dental prosthesis.

21: A range of 19th–century dentures.

22: A dental bridge designed to replace missing teeth.

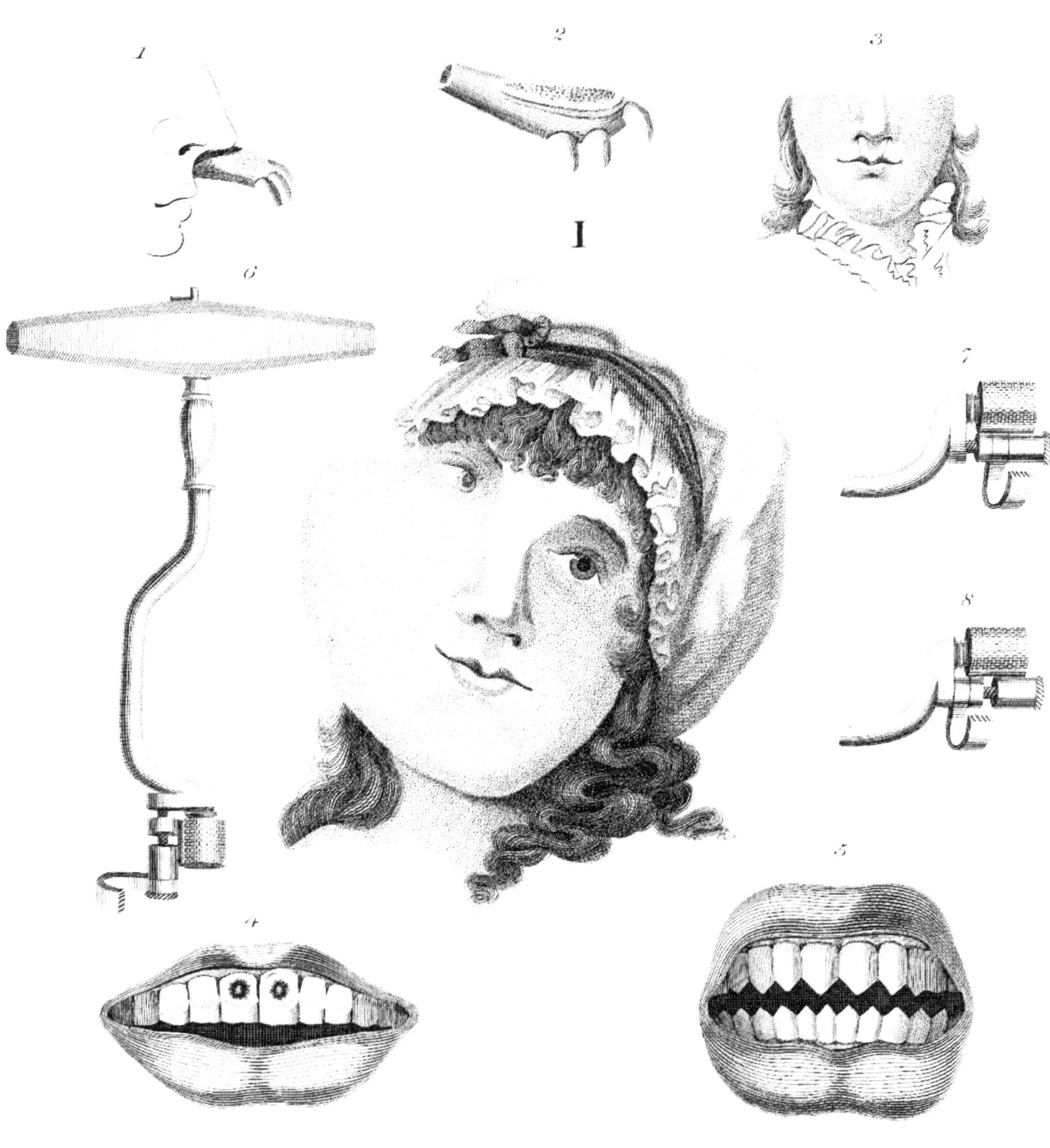




23: Various dental tools and teeth showing
defects.

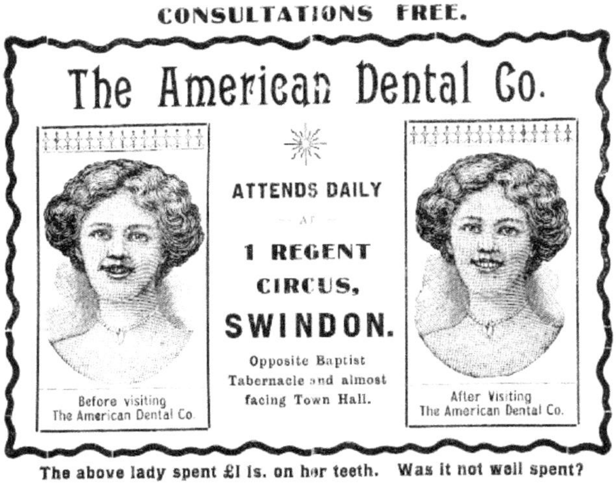

25

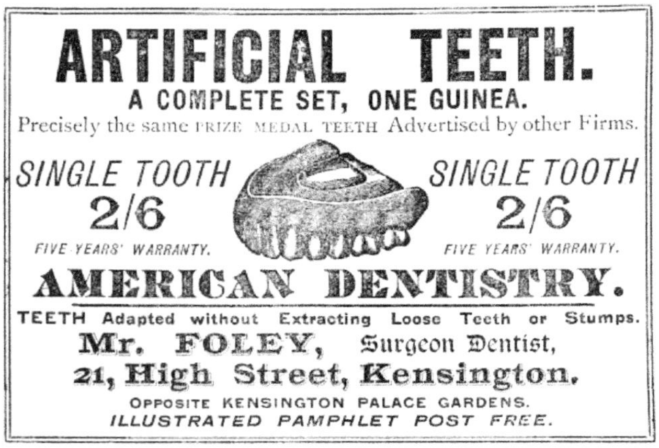

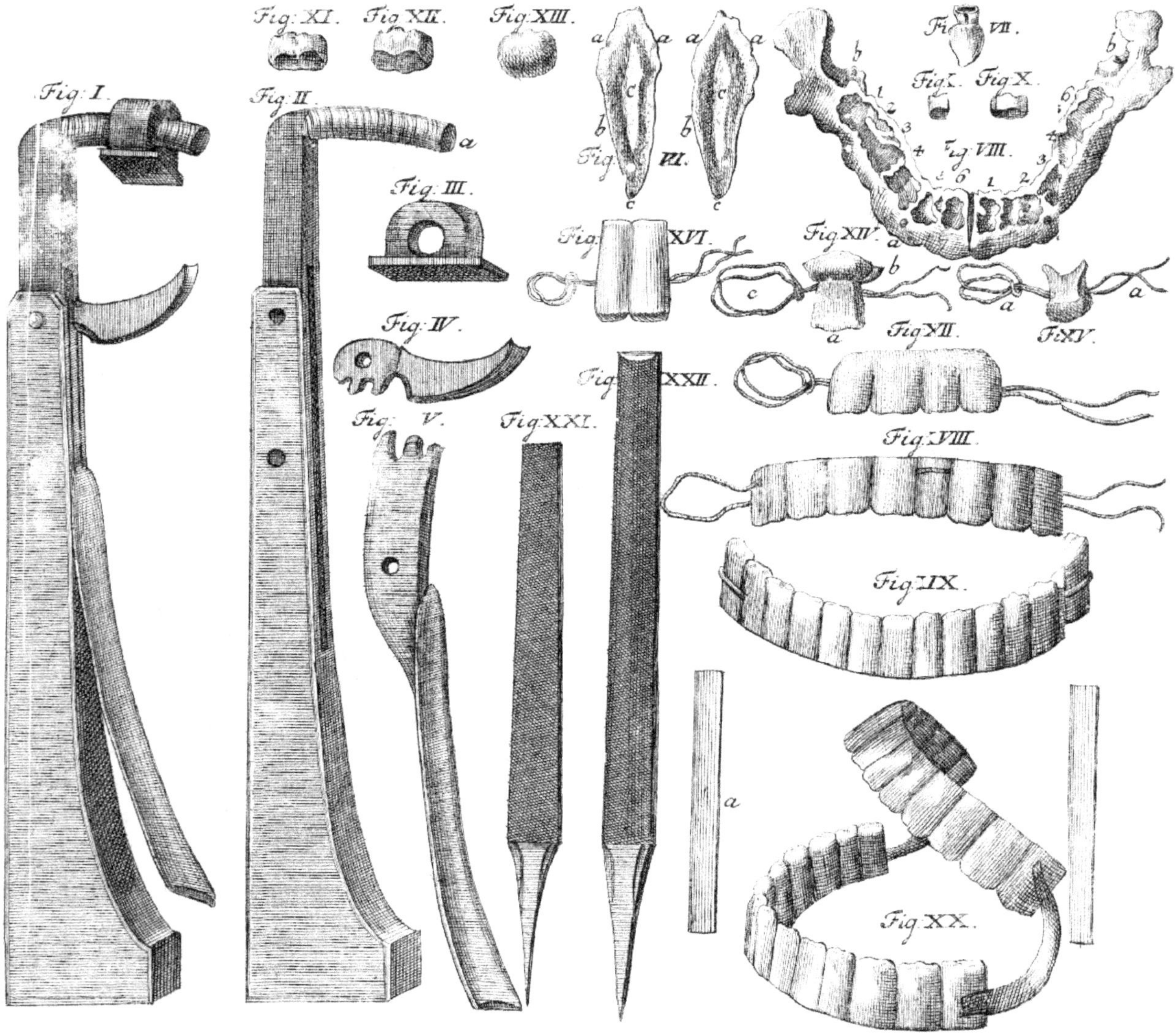

24: American Dentistry Advertisement.

25: Tools used for the construction of dental prosthesis.

26: American Dentistry Advertisement.

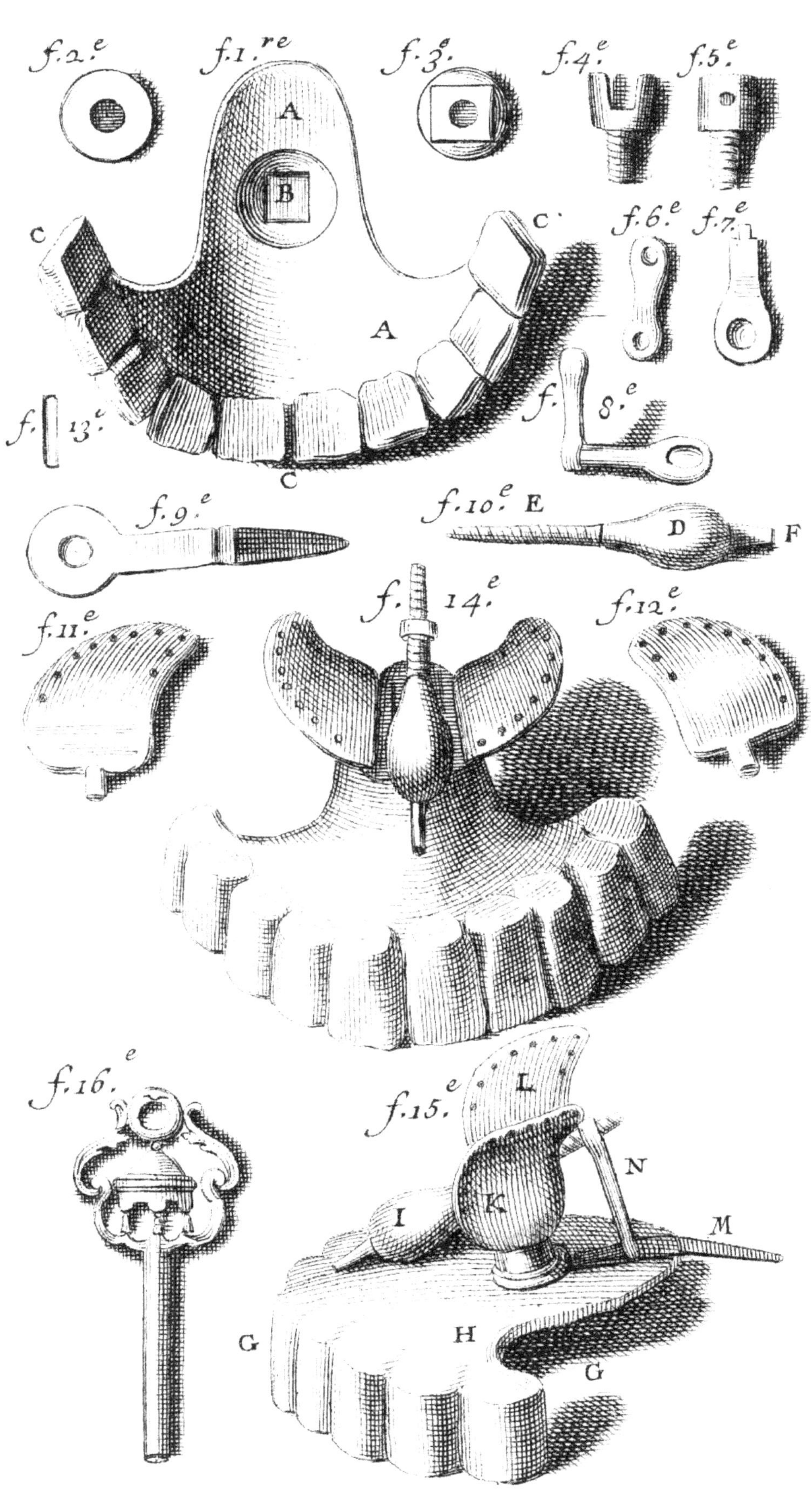


27: Tools used for the construction of dental prosthesis.

28



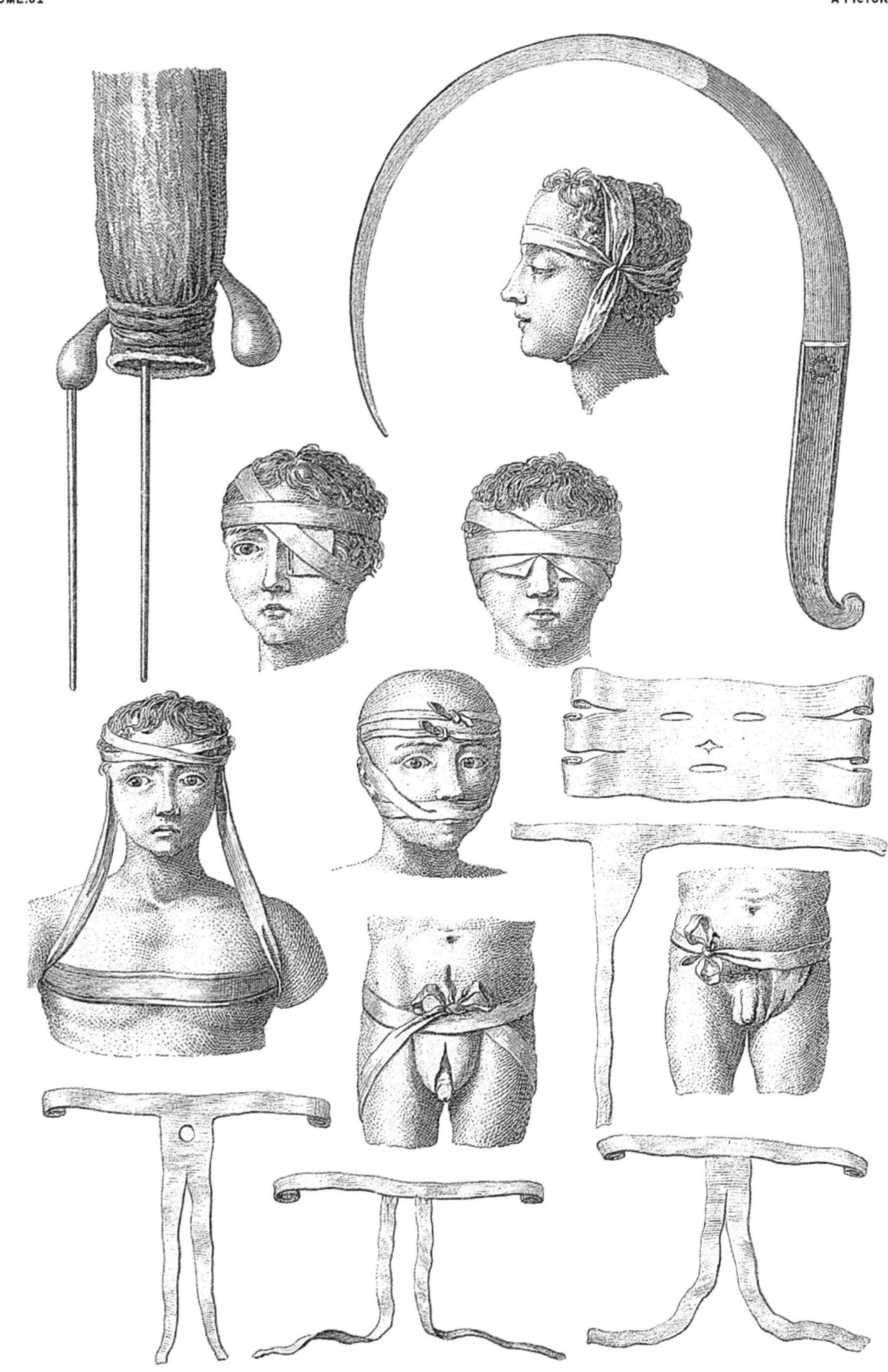

28: Top, an illustration of a rectum with a fistula;
below, a number of bandage techniques.

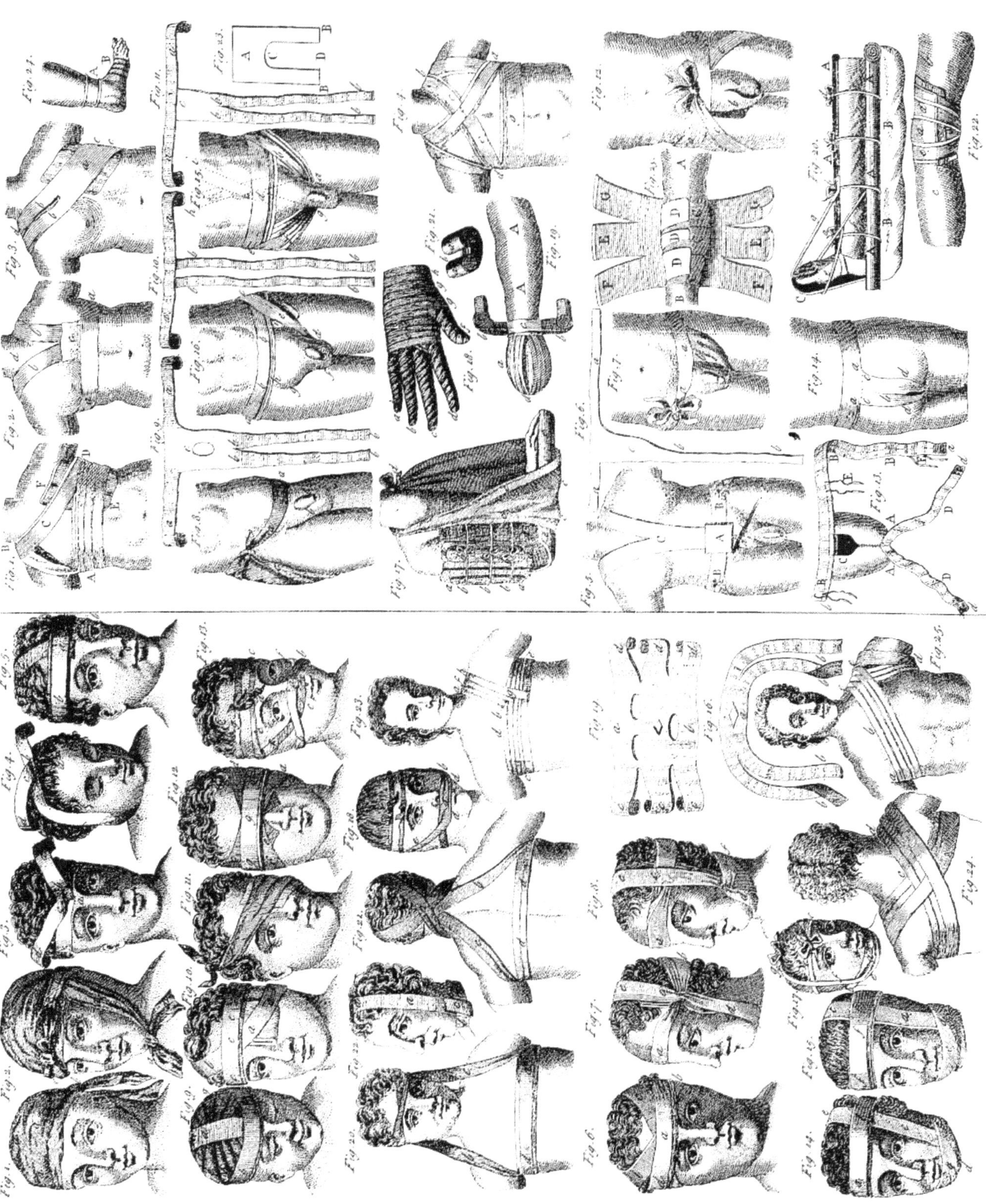



29: Surgical bandages and bandage applications.

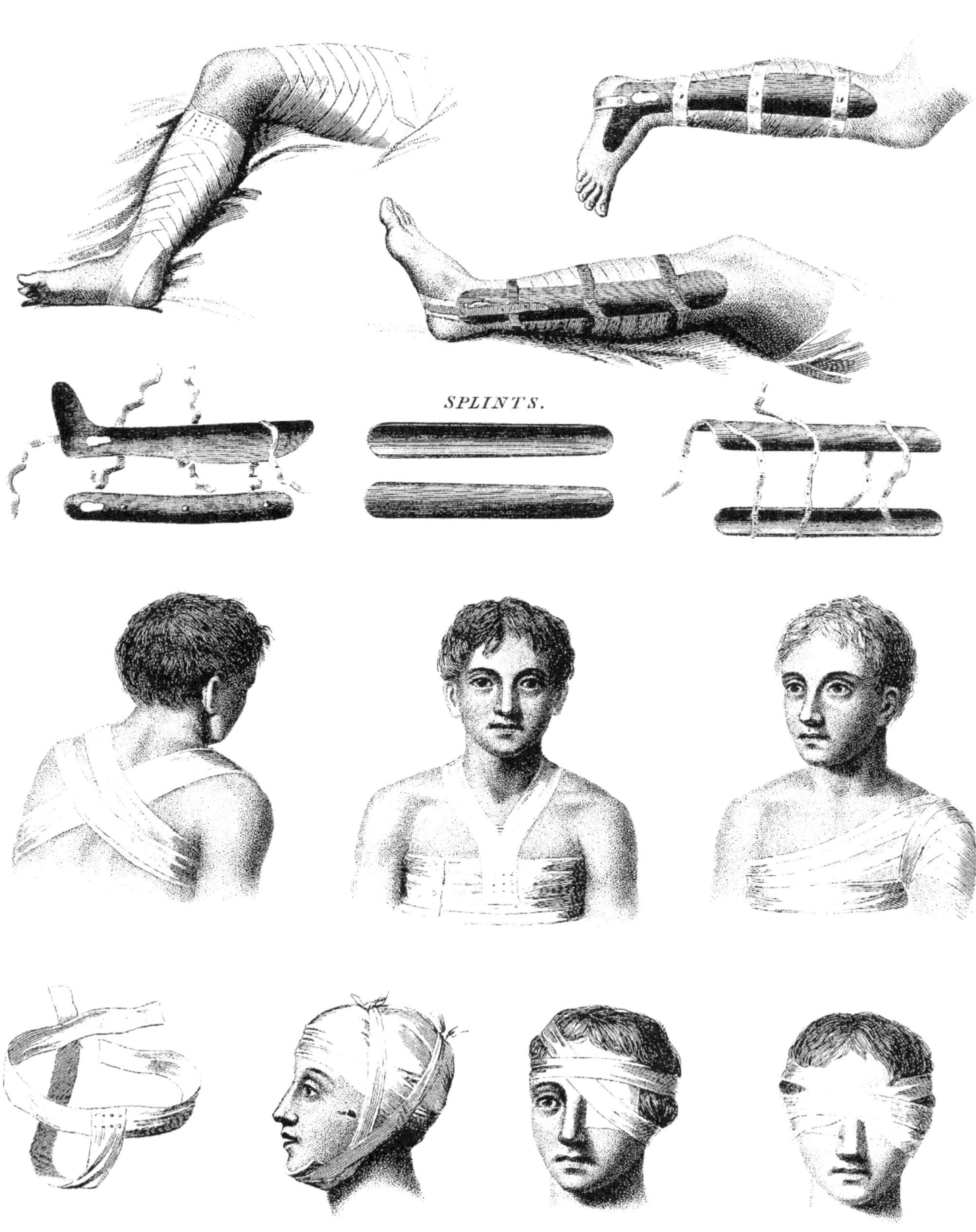


30: Fractured legs in splints, , bandages and
bandage applications.

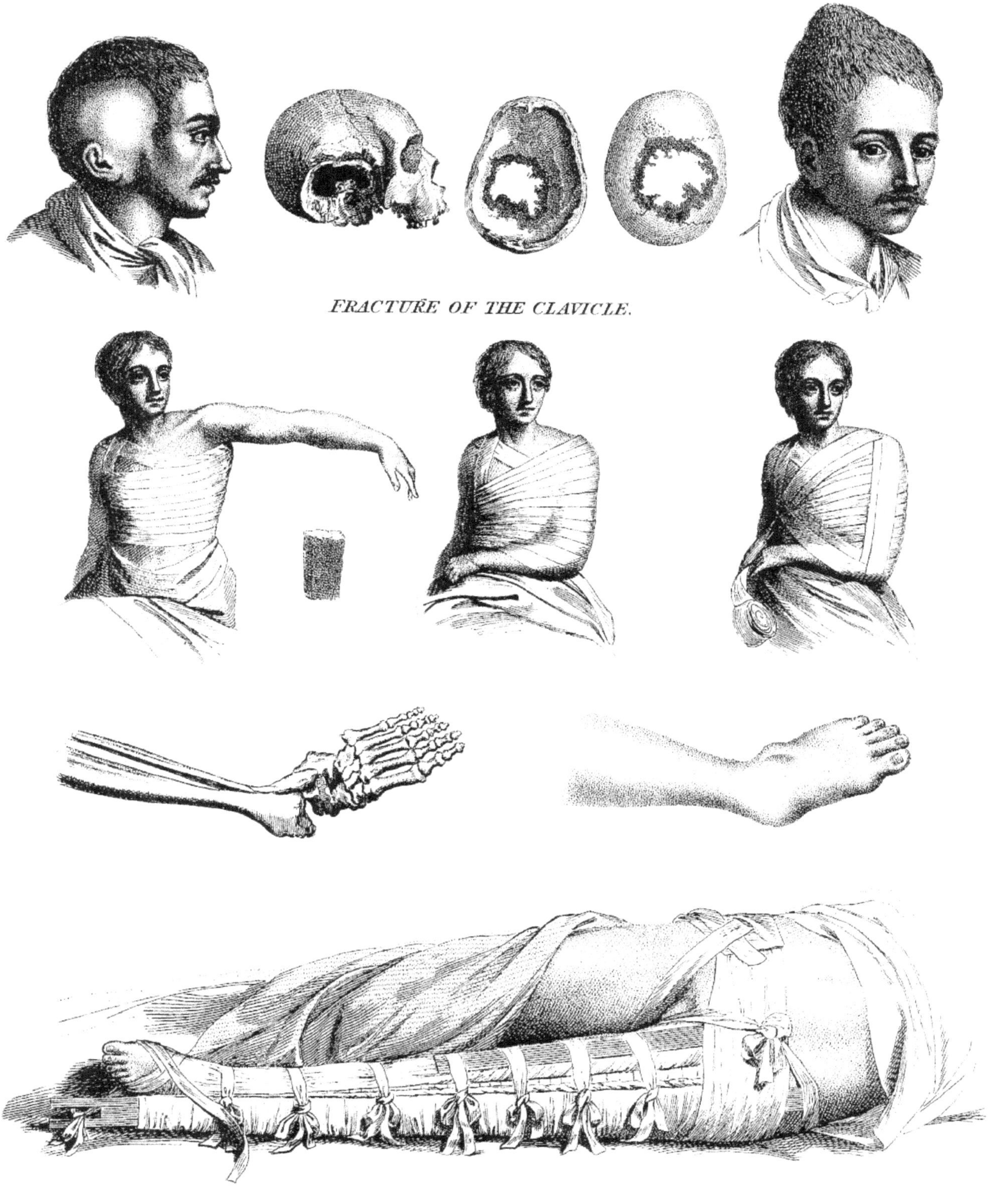

FRACTURE OF THE CLAVICLE.

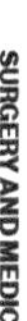
SURGERY AND MEDICINE

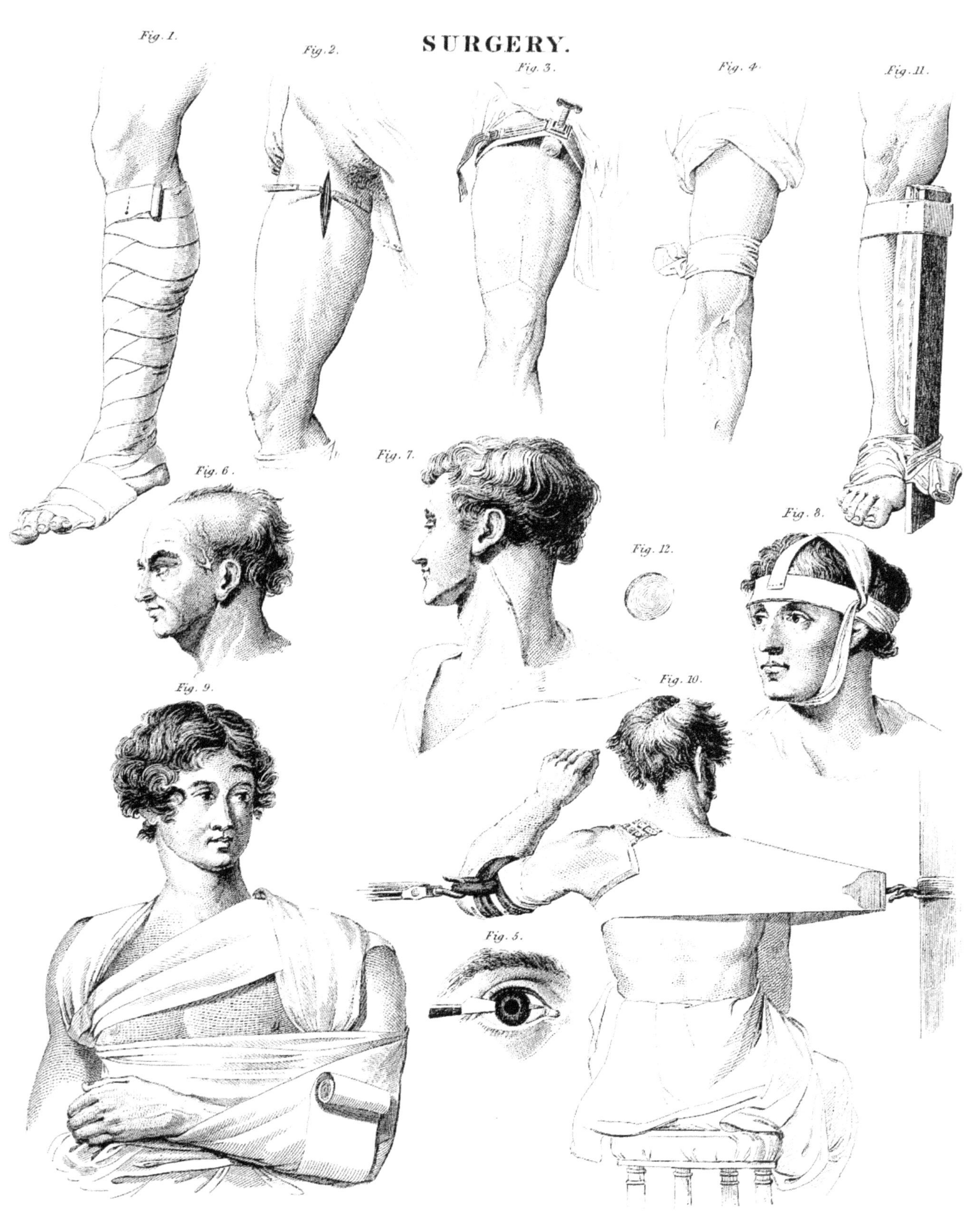


32: Bandaged legs with three with three various types of splints, heads showing
veins on the neck and temple, a bandaged head, a bandaged arm and torso, a
device for treating shoulder dislocations and a cataract operation.

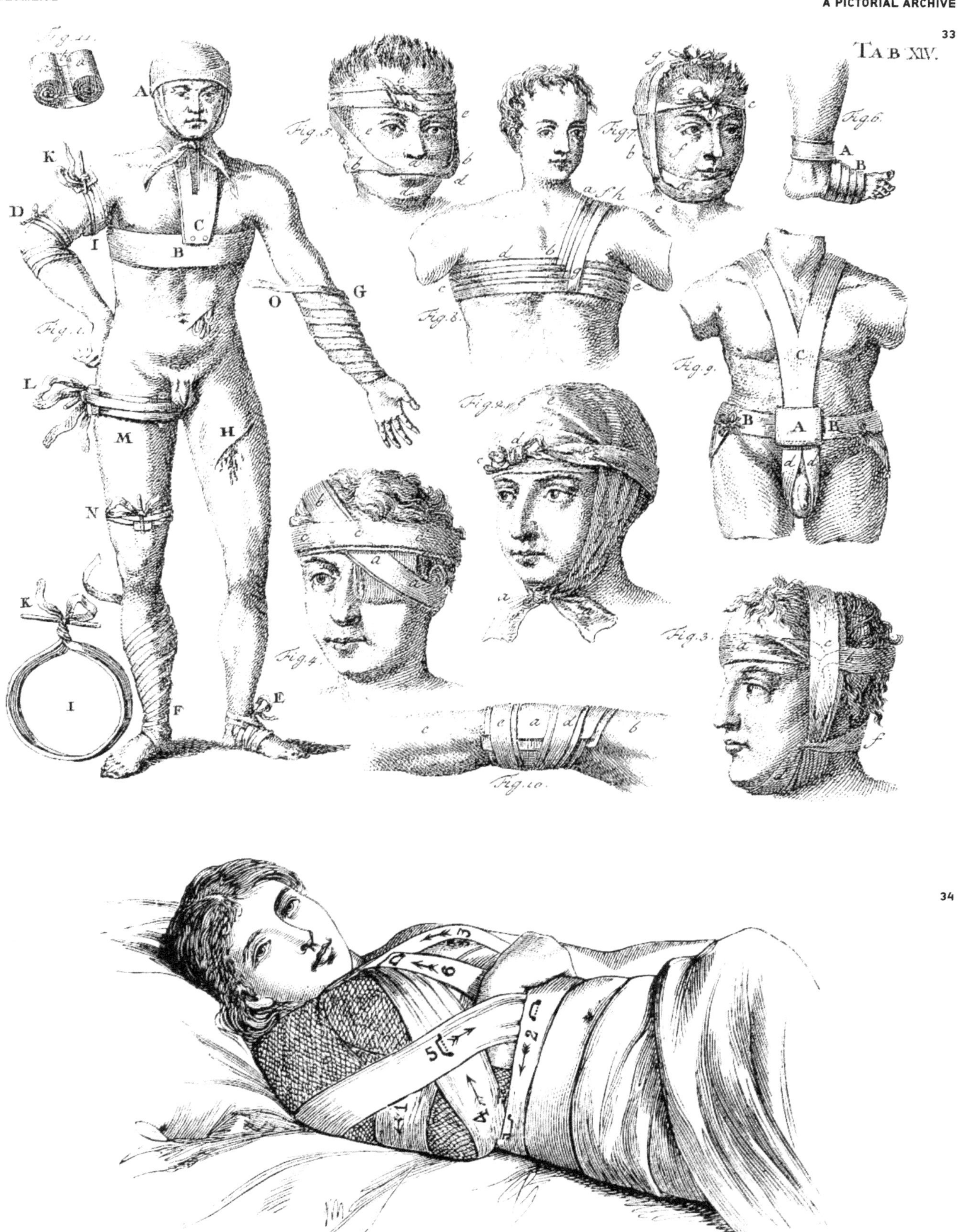



FIG. 41—DRESSINGS APPLIED AFTER EXCISION OF MAMMA AND AXILLARY GLANDS, TO SHOW THE ARRANGEMENT OF THE DRESSINGS AND BANDAGES.



33: Various applications of bandages to the head, breast, torso and leg.

34: Dressings applied after excision of mamma and axillary glands.

35



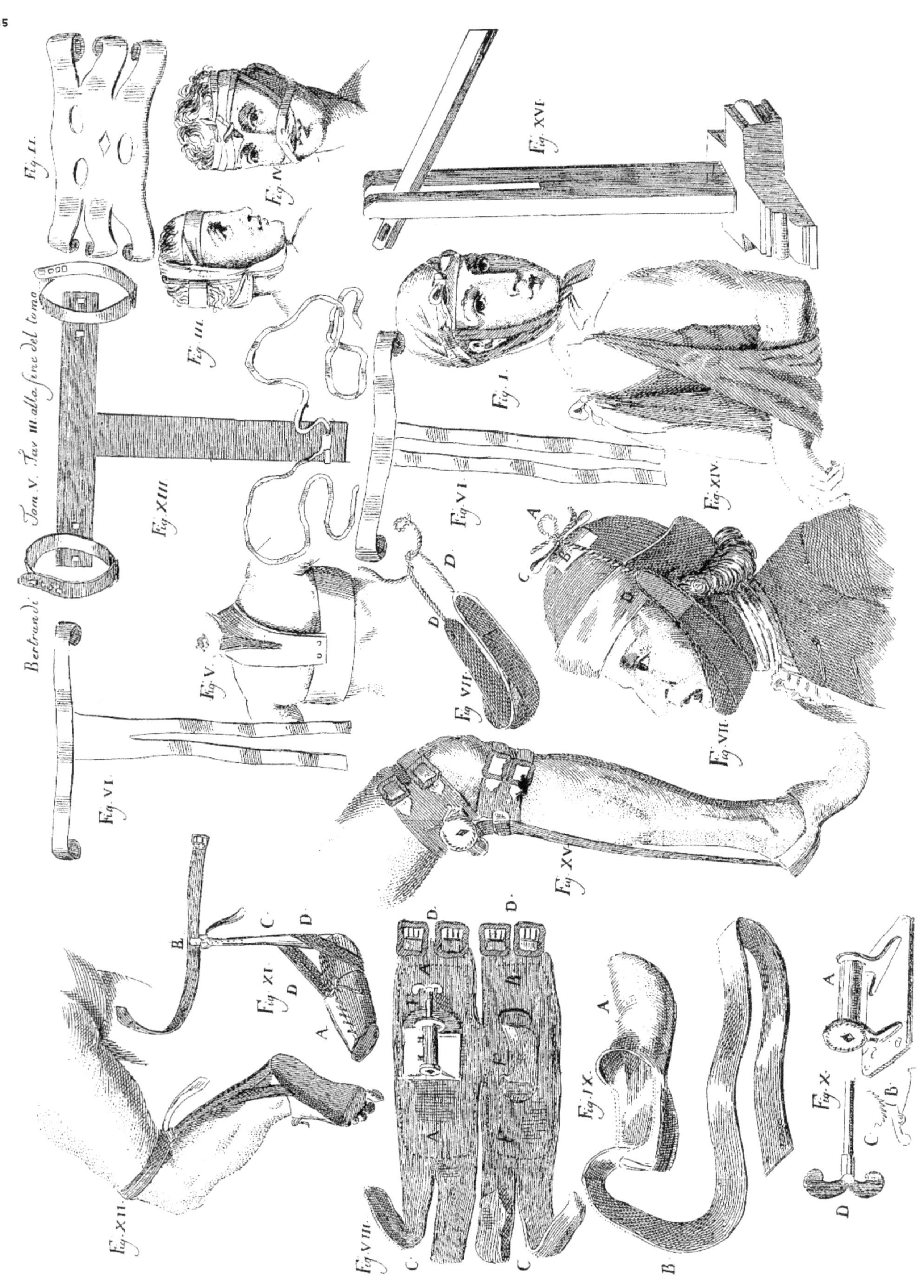

35: Bandages from Bertrandi's 'Opere'.

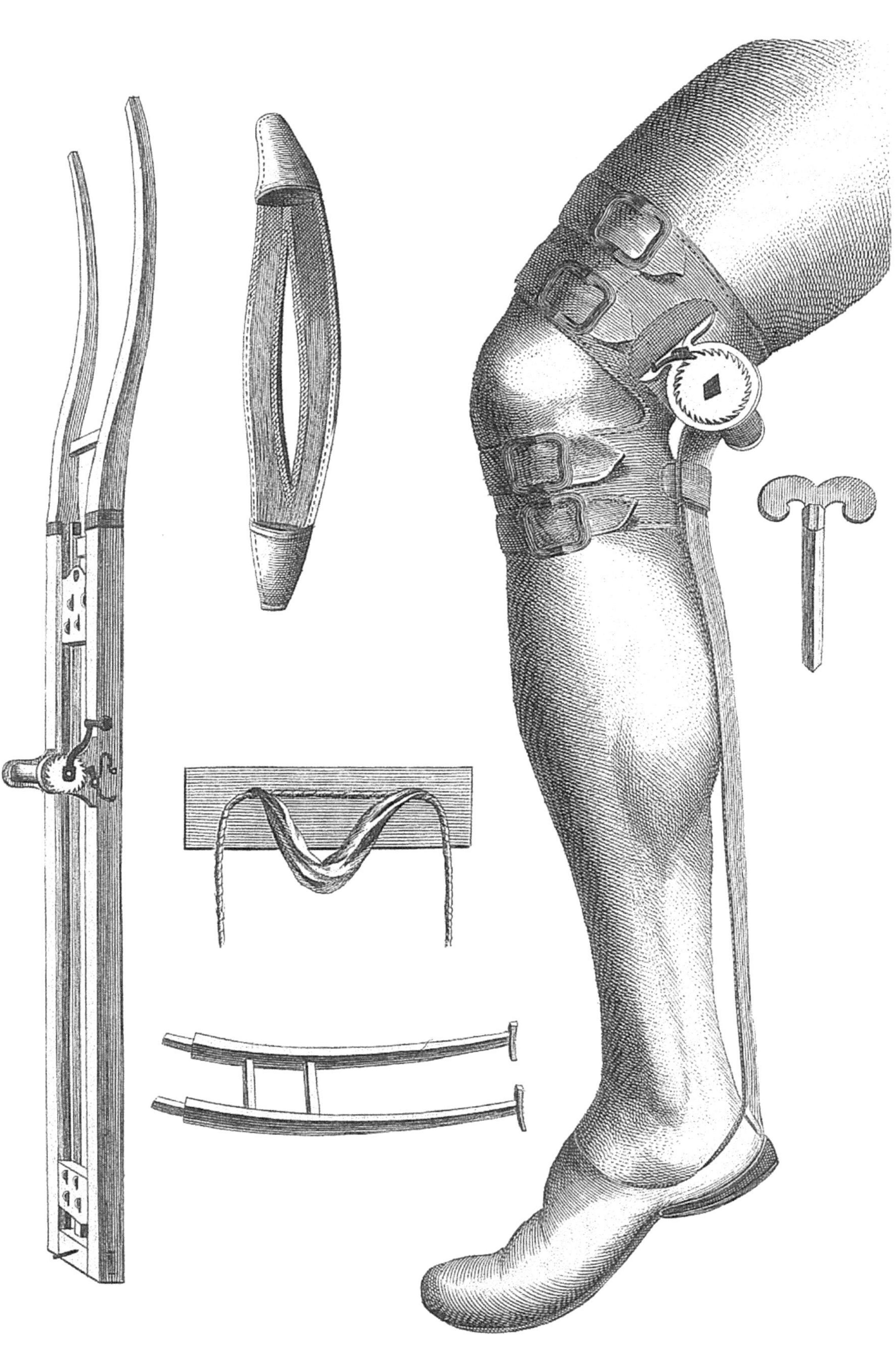



36: Surgical instruments used for the correction
of dislocated limbs.

37

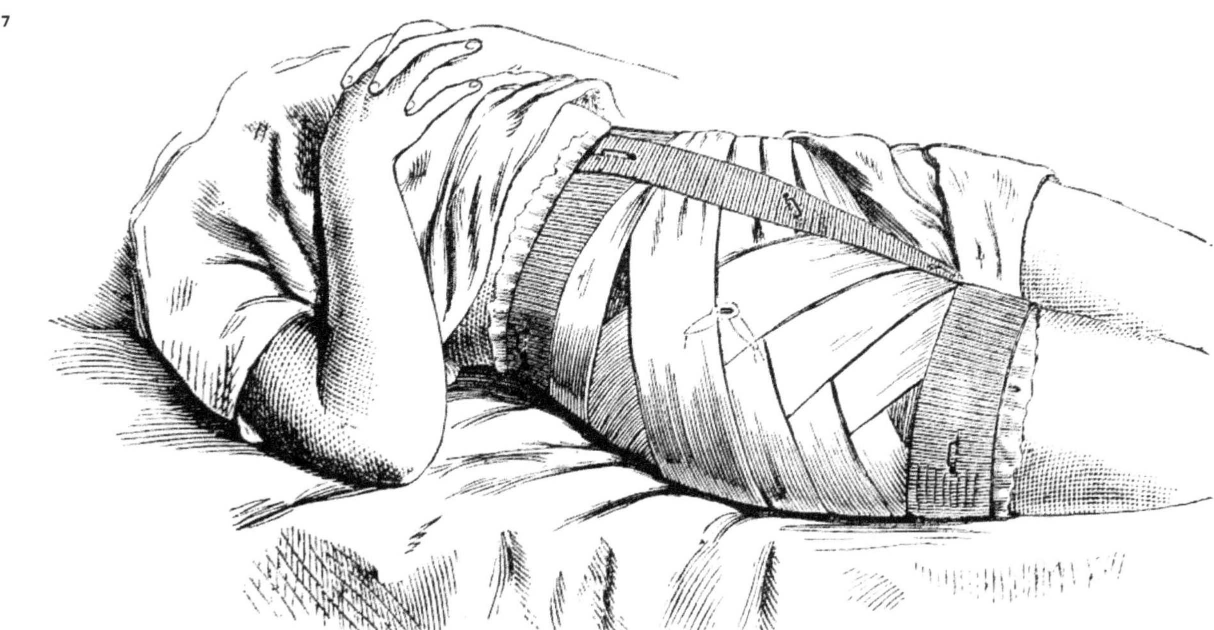

FIG. 37.—DRESSING IN A CASE OF PSOAS ABSCESS OPENED ABOVE
POUPART'S LIGAMENT.

To show the arrangement of the elastic bandage along the margins of the dressing.



38

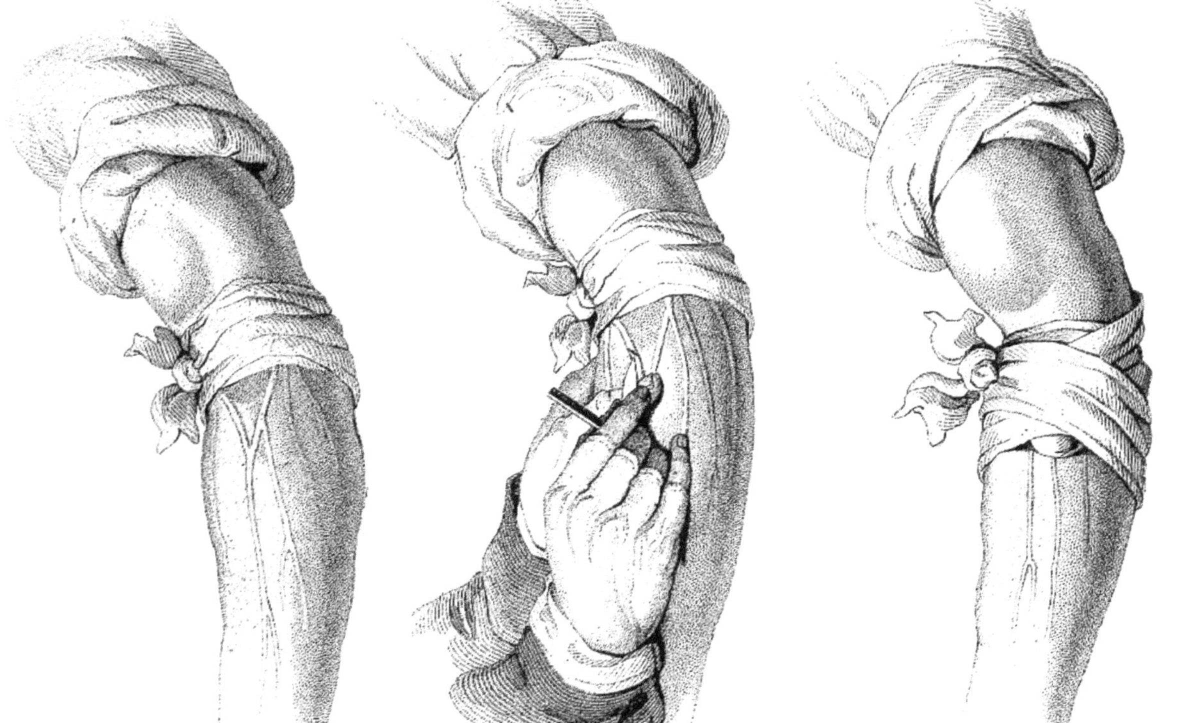


37: Dressing in a case of psoas abscess opened
above Poupart's ligament.

38: Three illustrations demonstrating blood
letting.

# FRACTURES

*PLATE III*

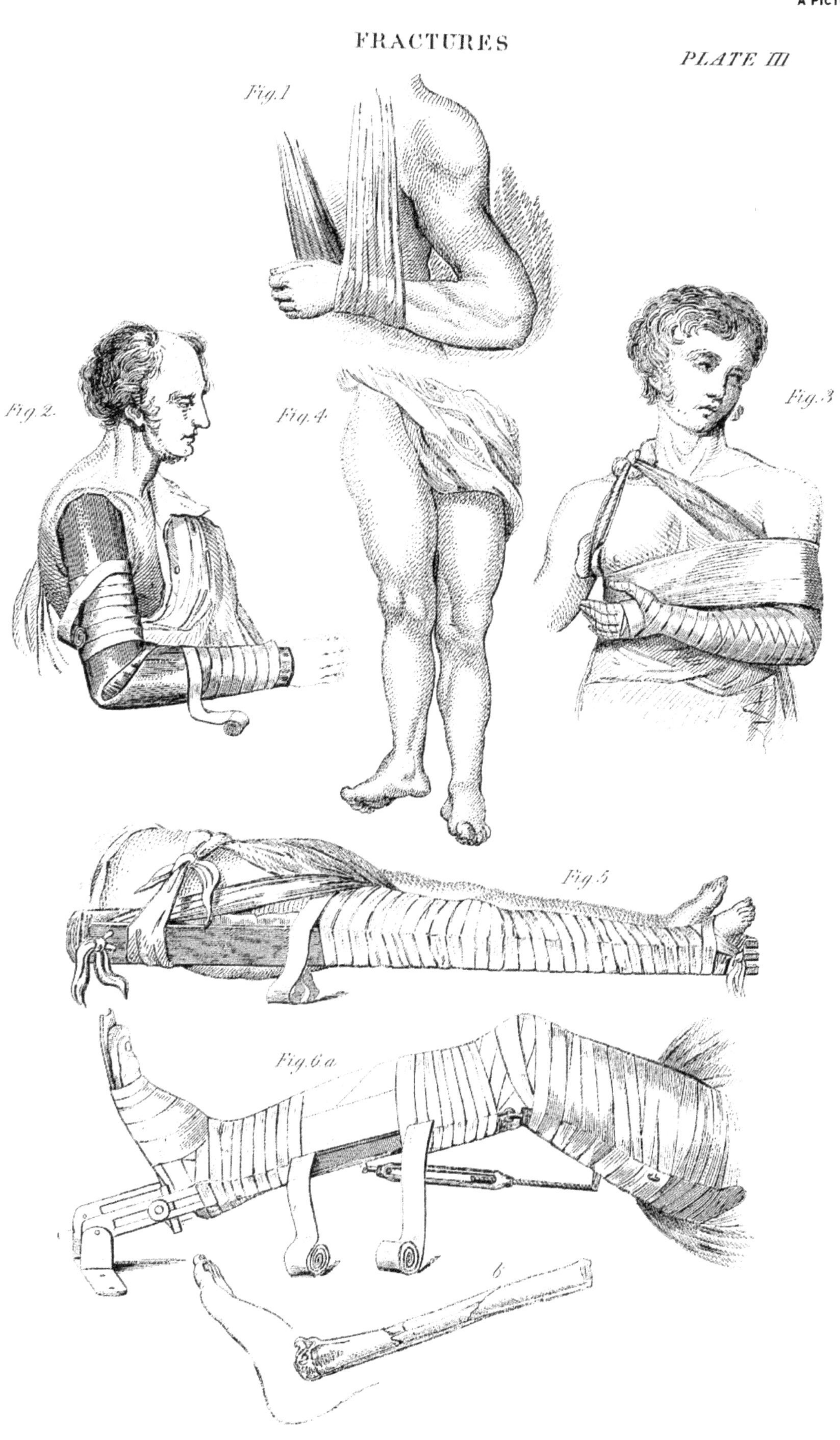




39: Diagrams illustrating how to bandage and set
fractured legs and arms with splints.

40



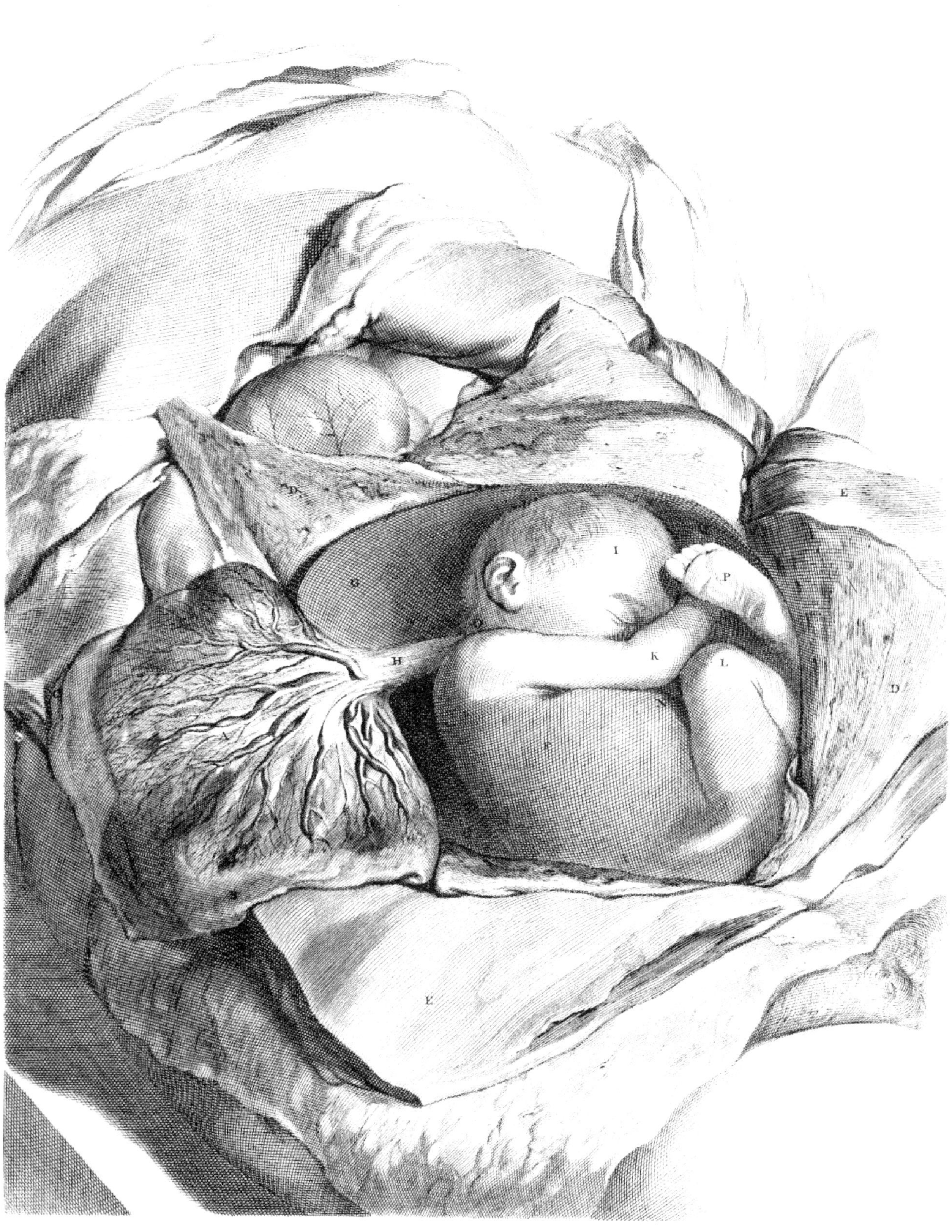

40: Anatomical study of the inside of the uterus
and a foetus.

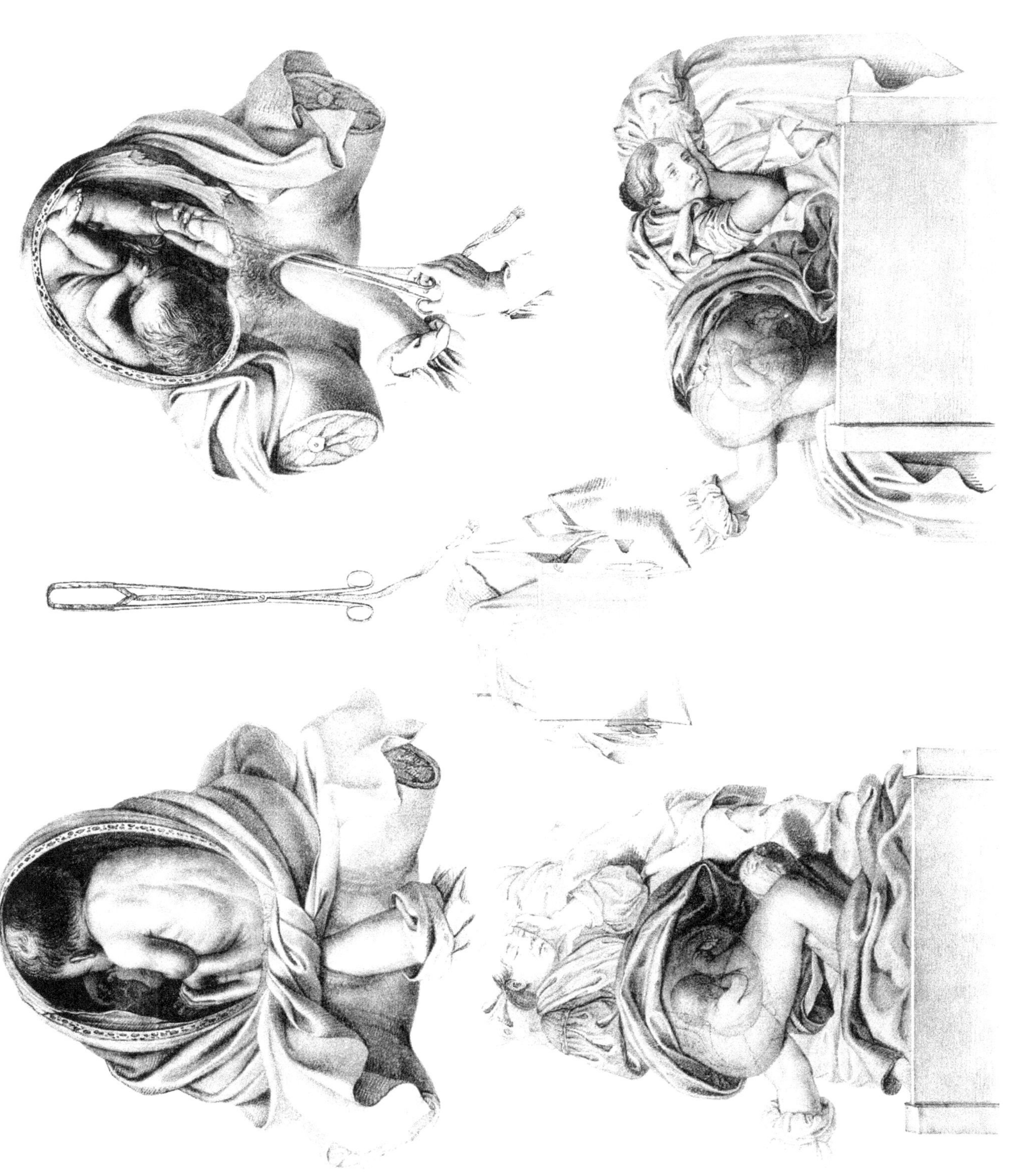

41: Breech presentation.

42

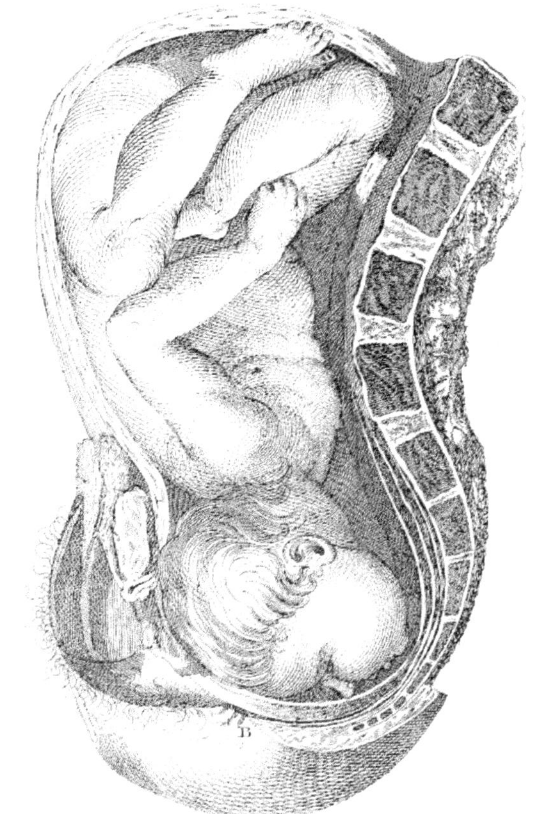

44

43

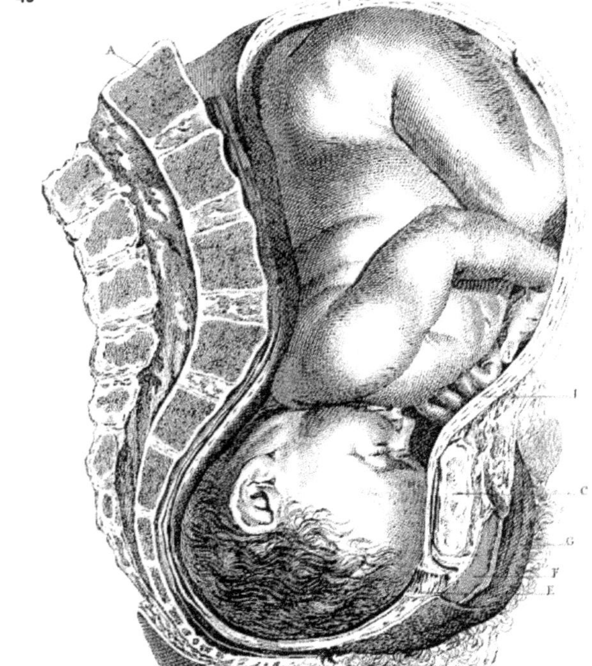

45

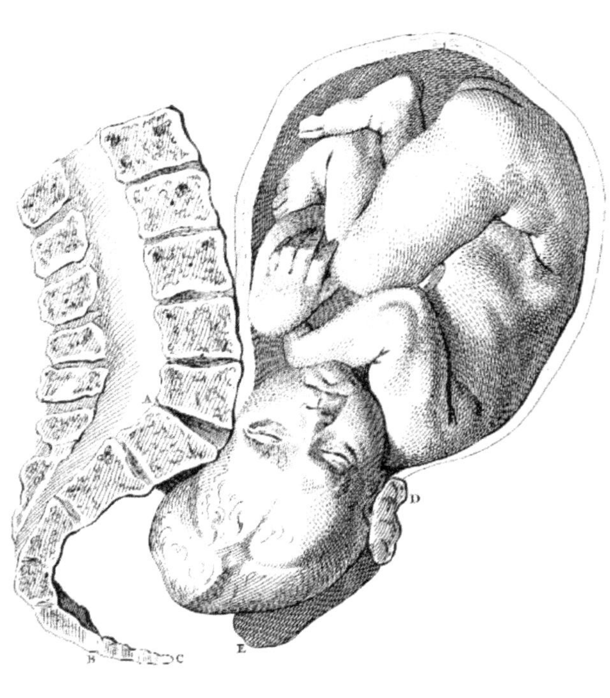

42 – 45: Illustrations show a foetus in utero.

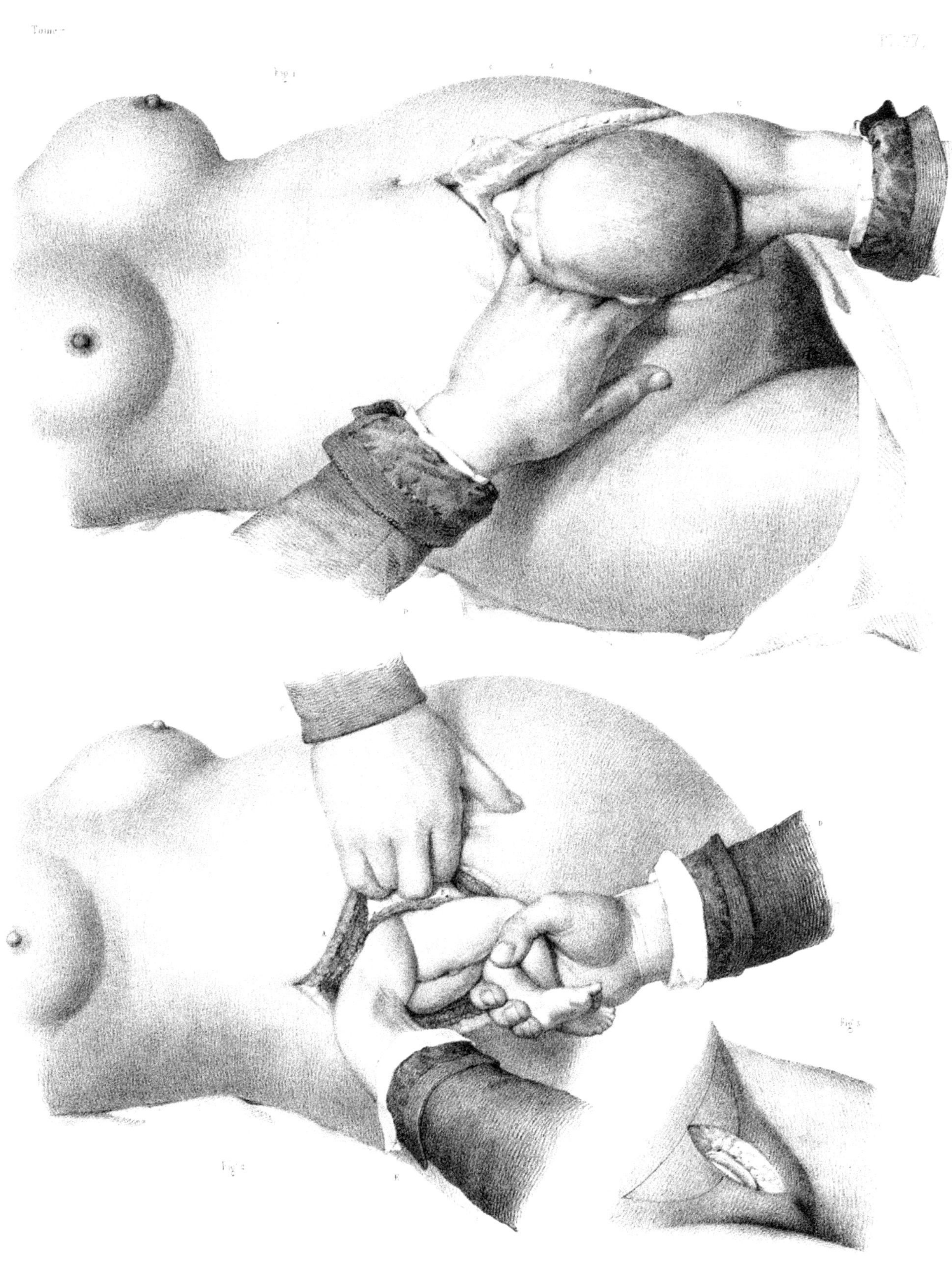

46: Delivery by caesarean section.

47



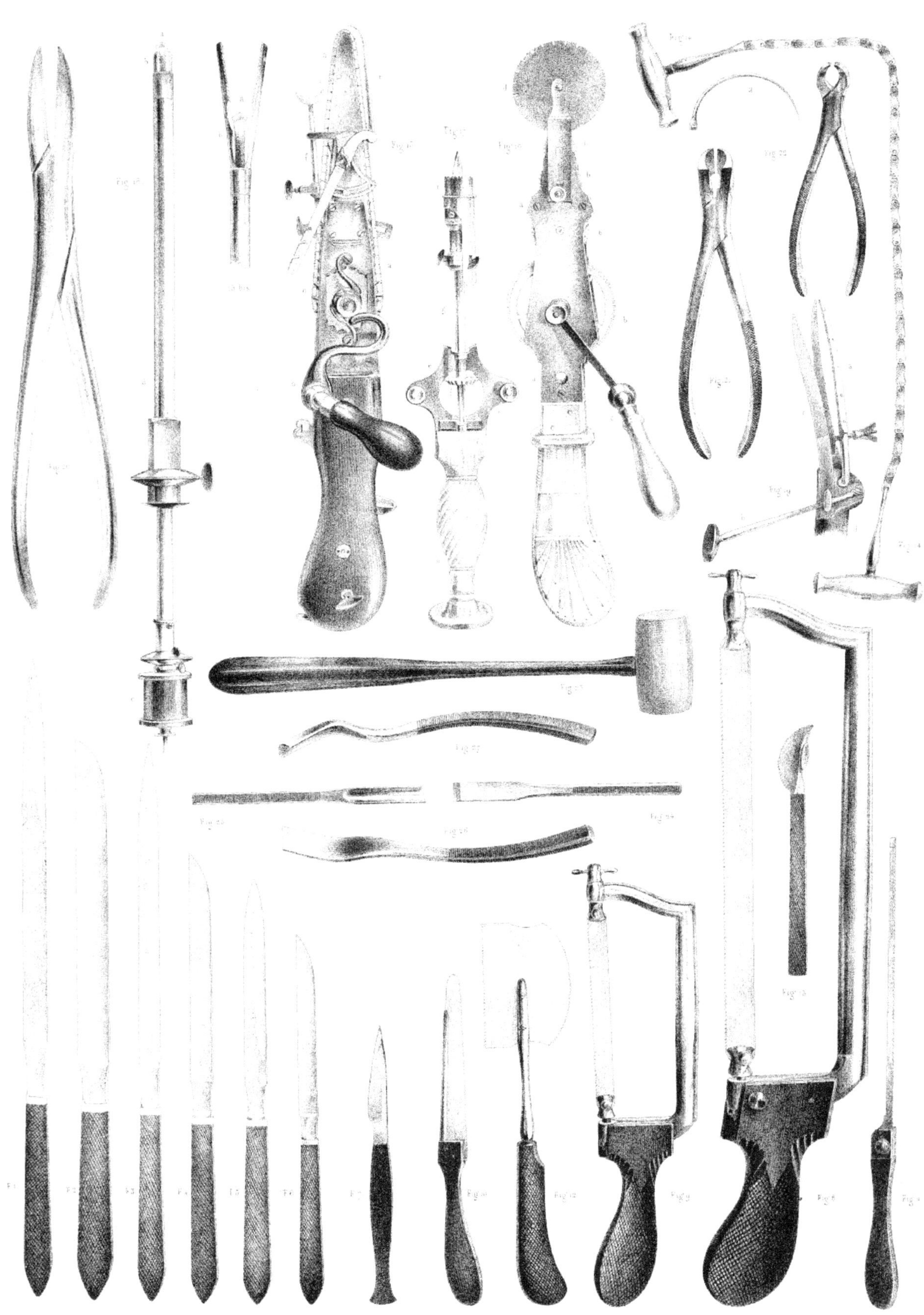

47: Surgical instruments for operating on bones.

48

49

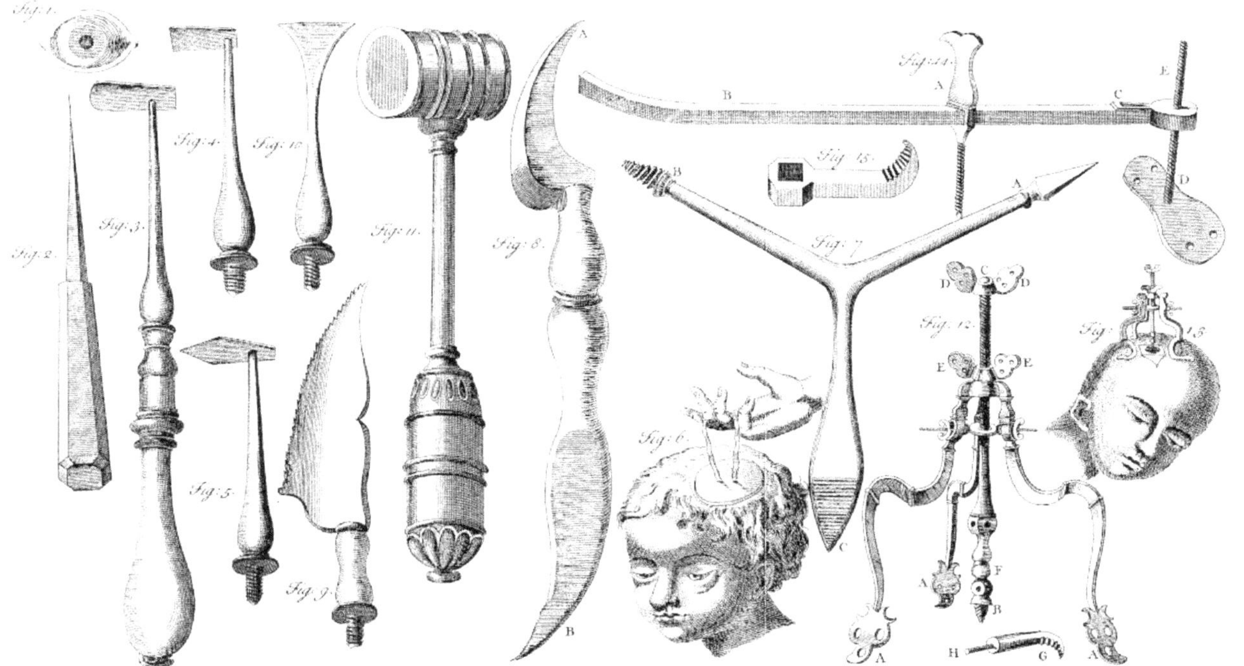

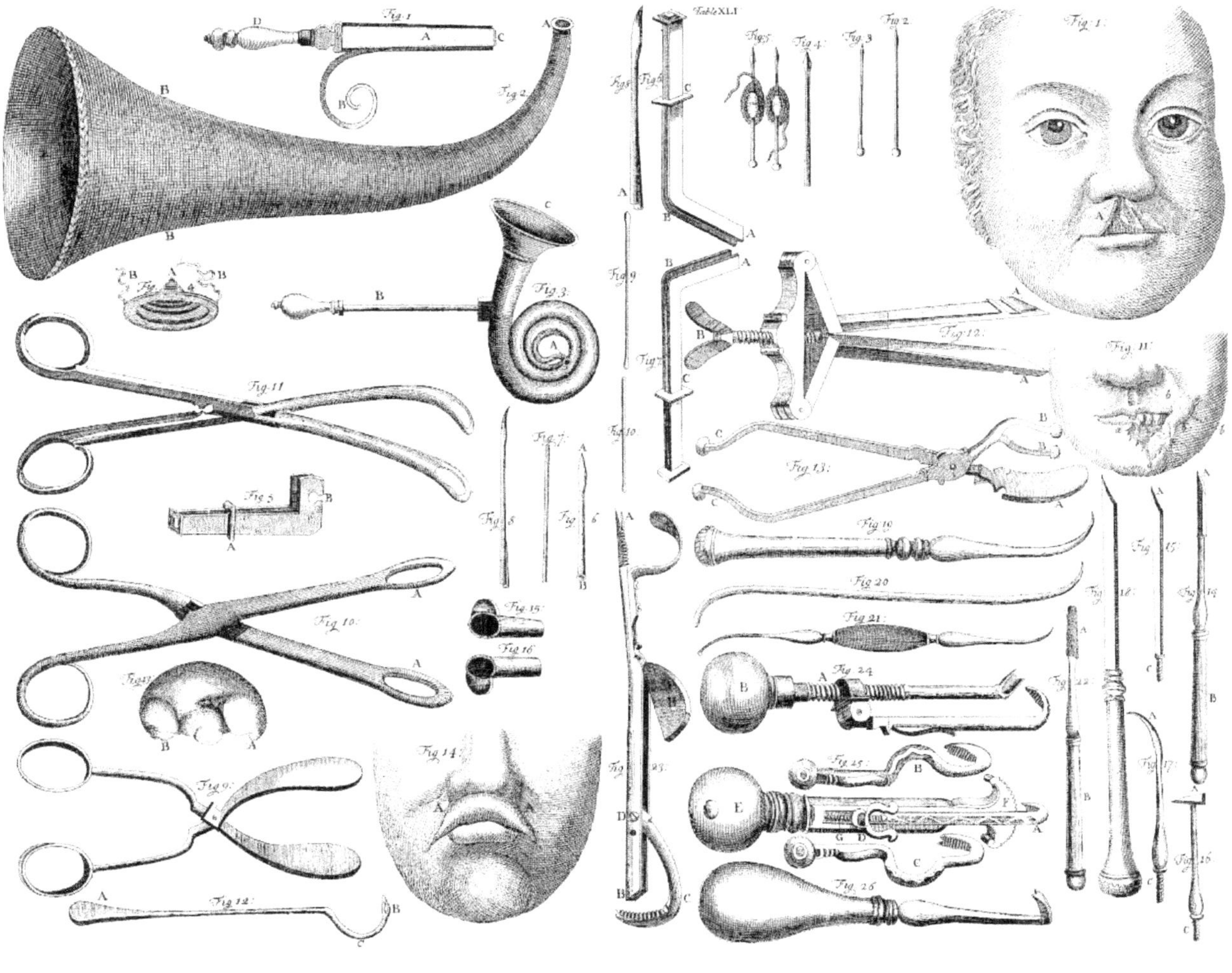

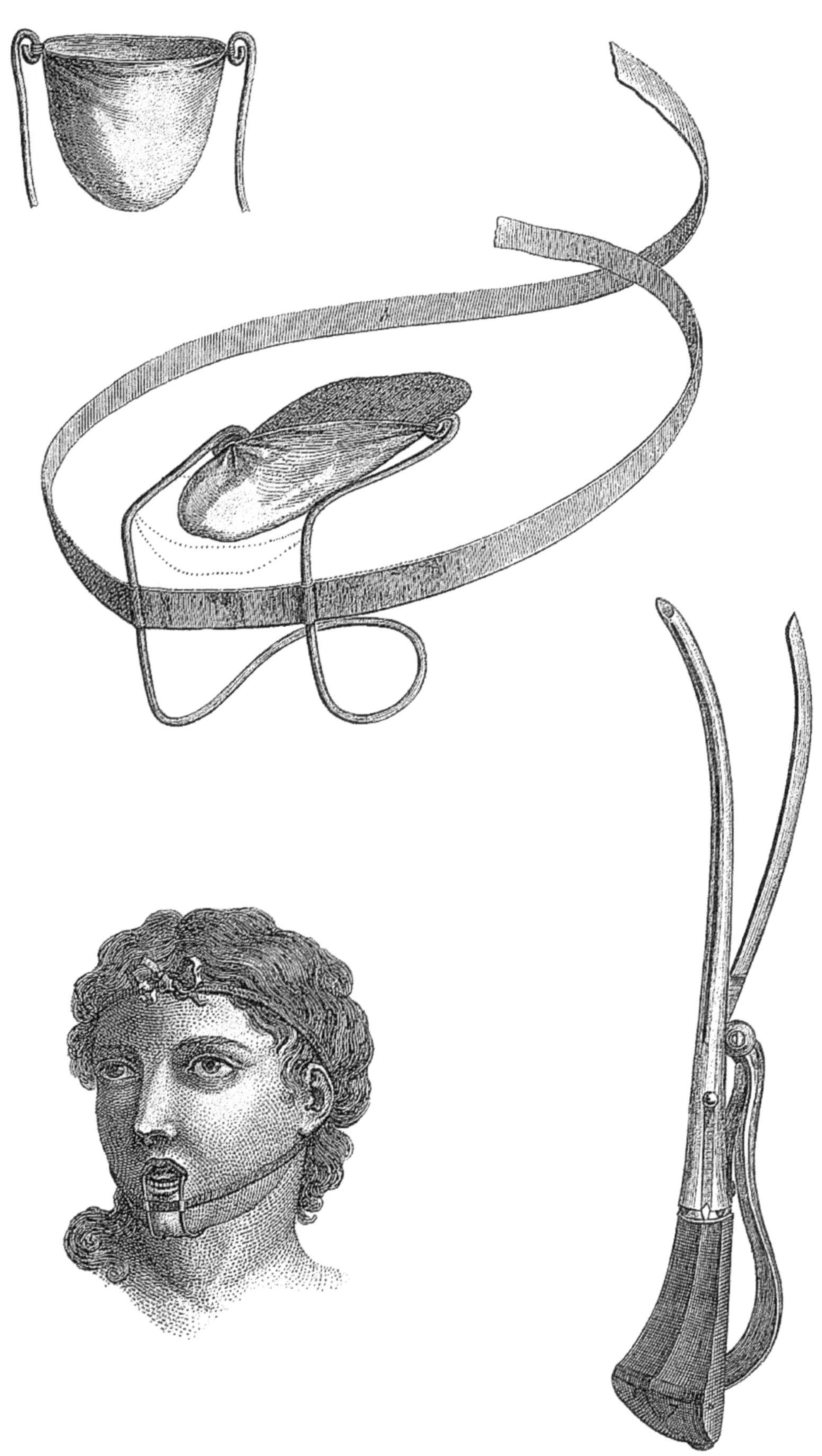



50



50: Surgical instruments and a dressing for
the tongue.

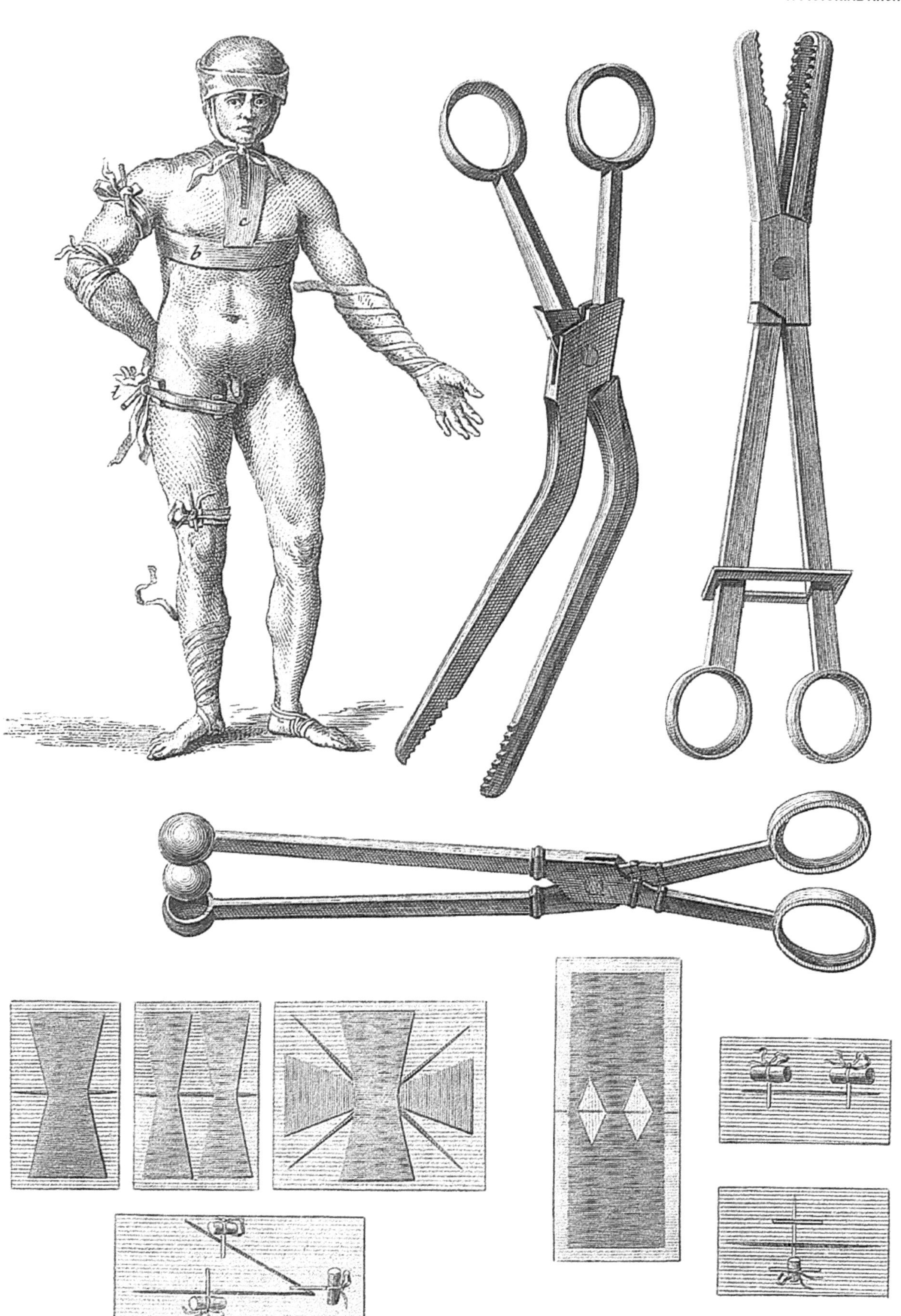



51: Surgical instruments and varying techniques
for surgical sutures.

52

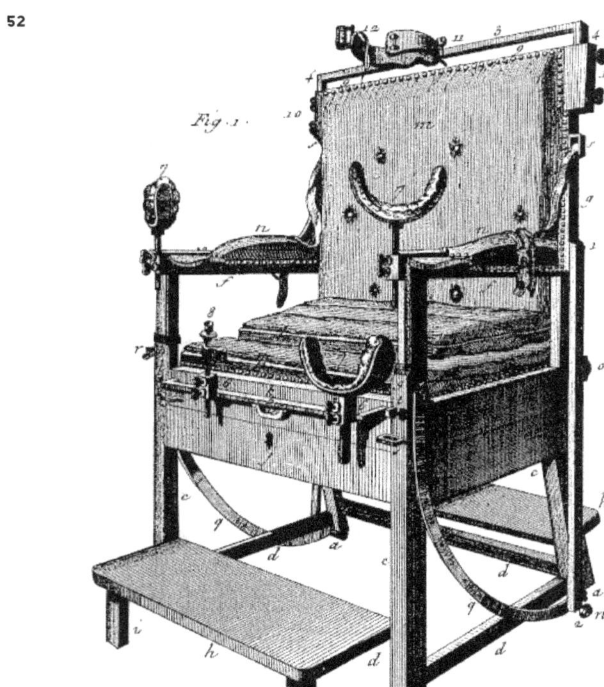
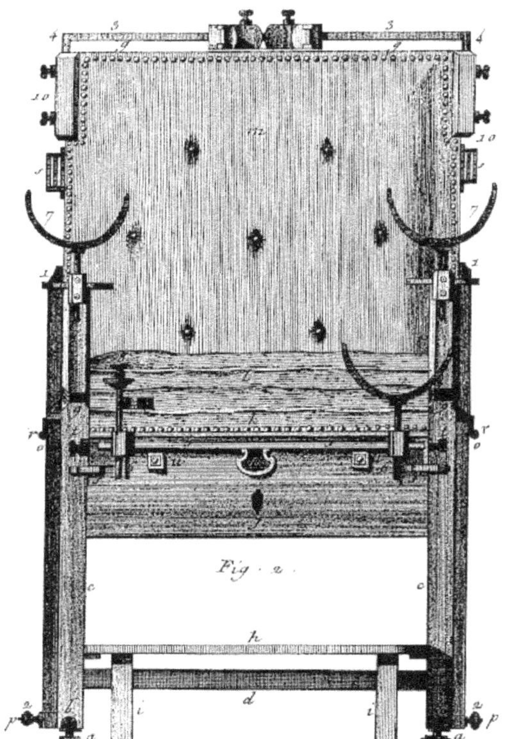



53

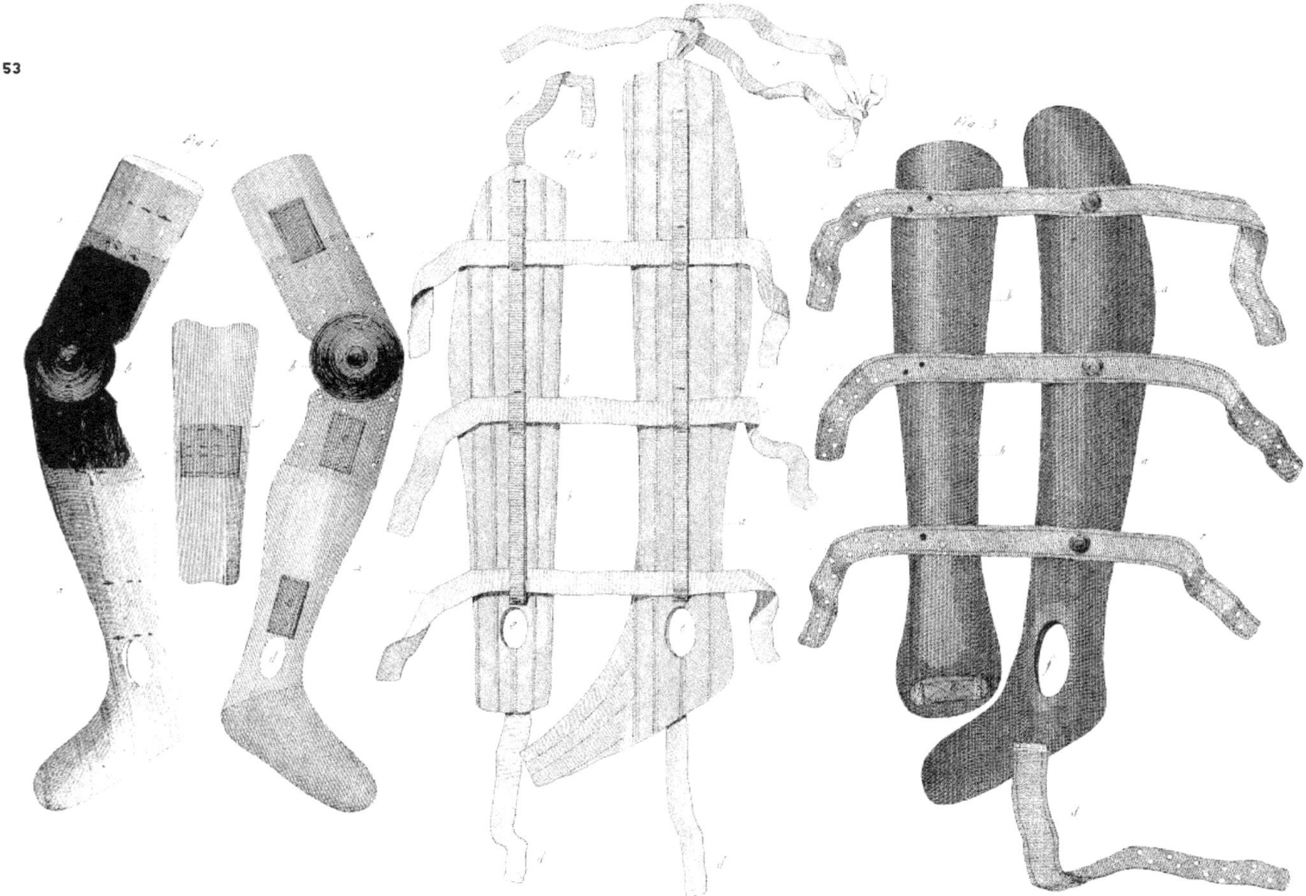

52: Surgical chairs.

53: Three different types of surgical splints.

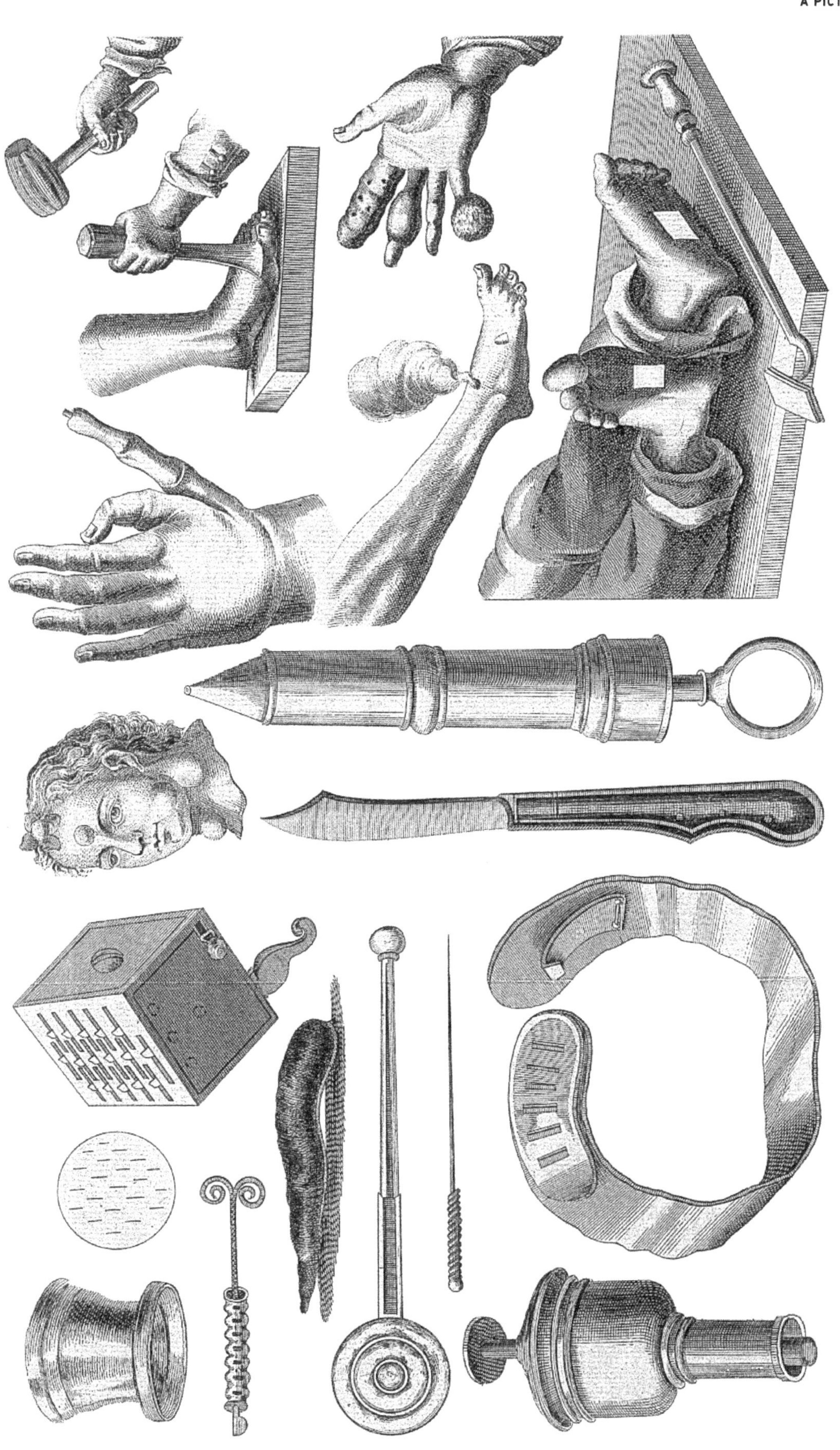



54: Surgical instruments.

55

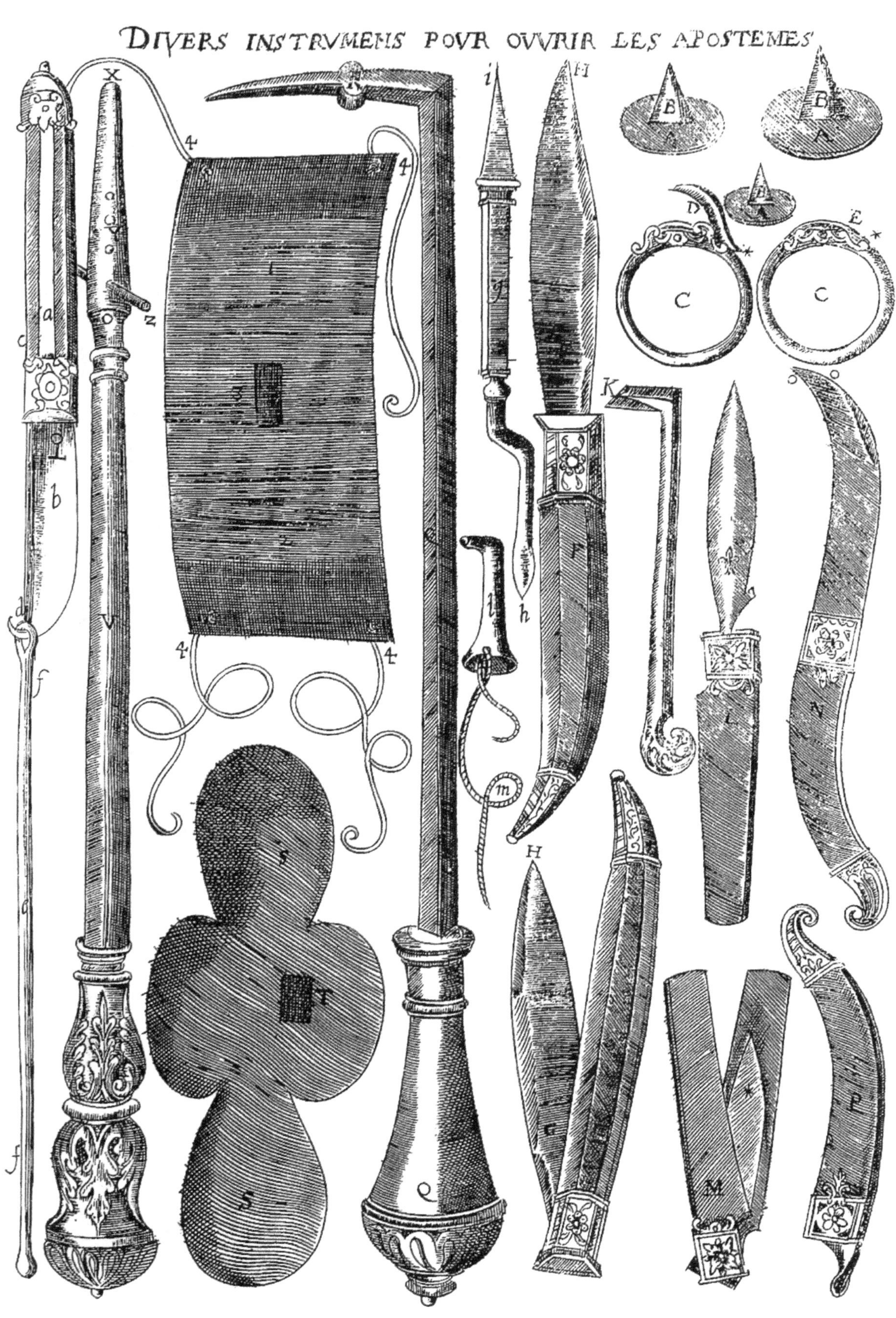


55: Knives and lancets for removal of abscesses.

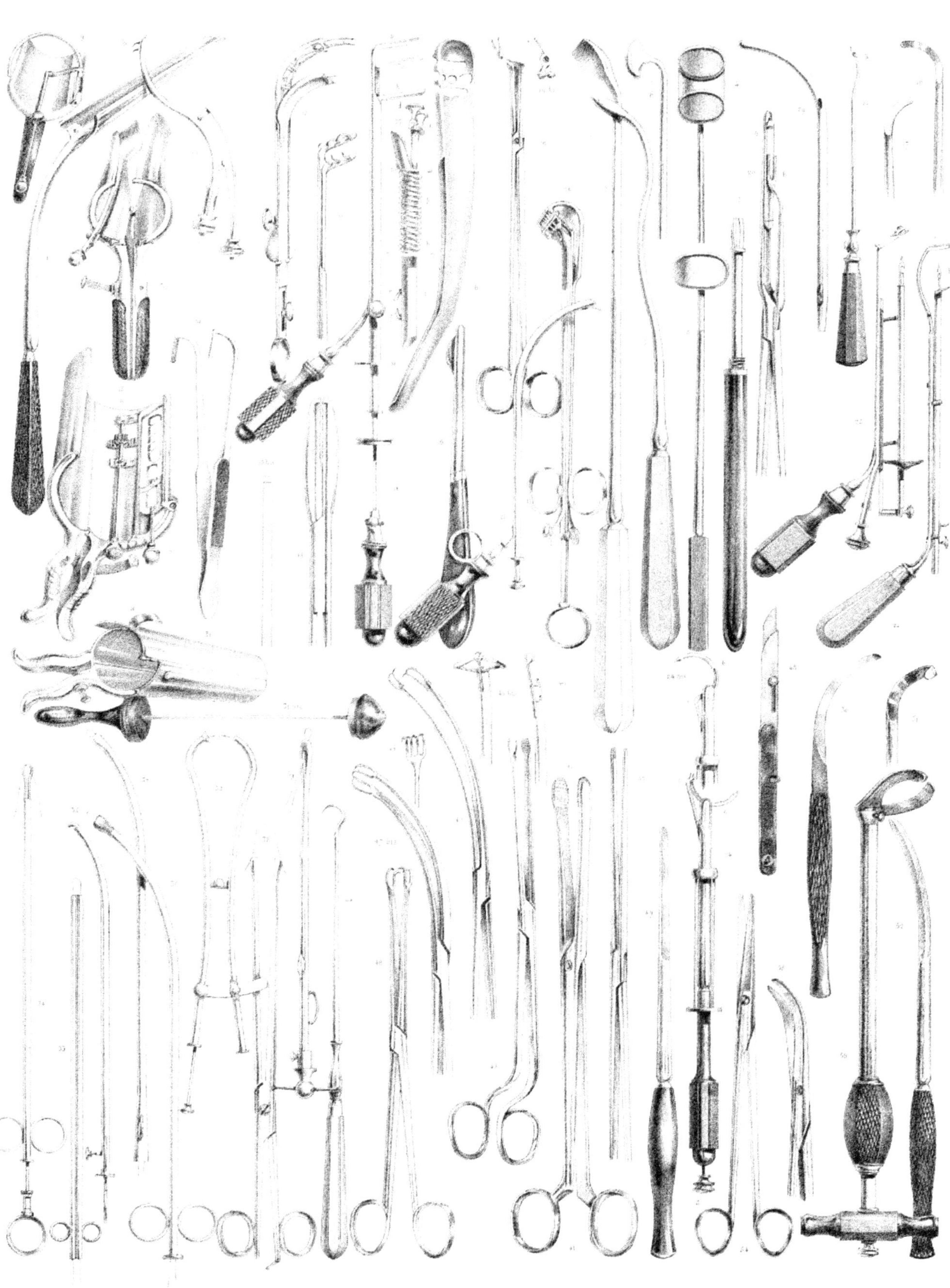



56: Surgical instruments for use on female
reproductive organs.

57



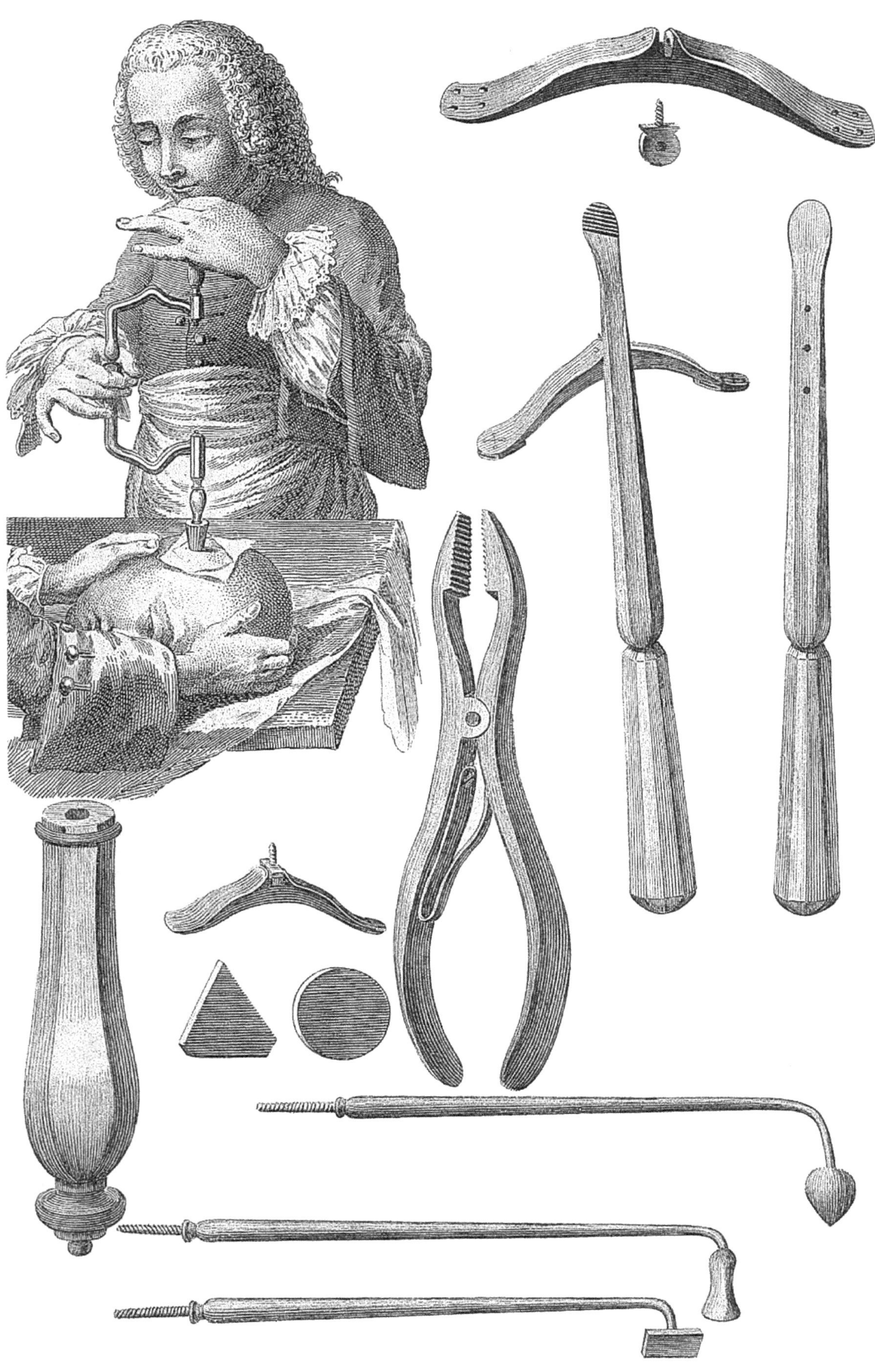

57: A skull being trepanned by a surgeon; below,
various instruments used for trepanation.

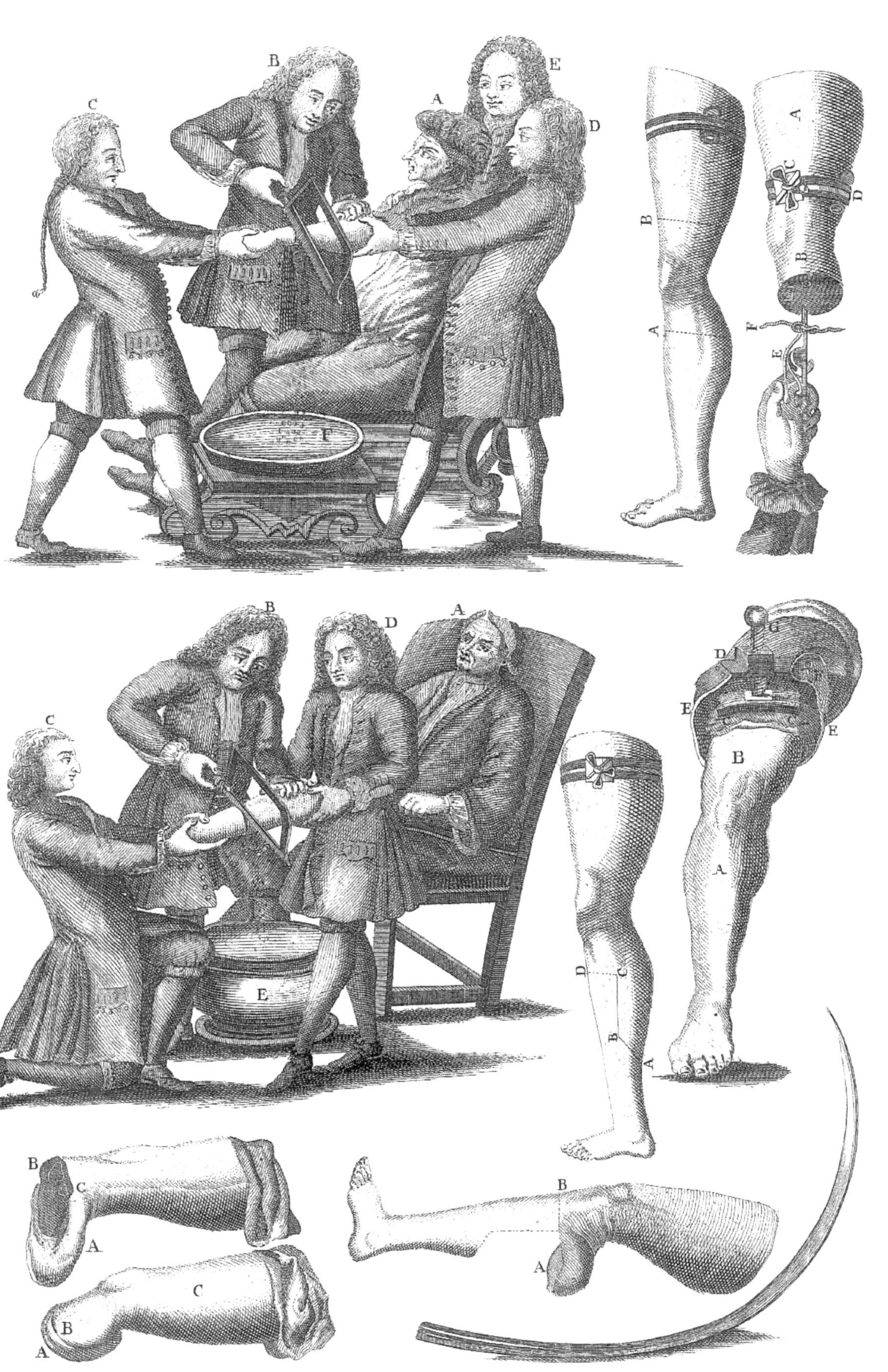



58: Amputations of arm and leg with process
diagrams.

59



60

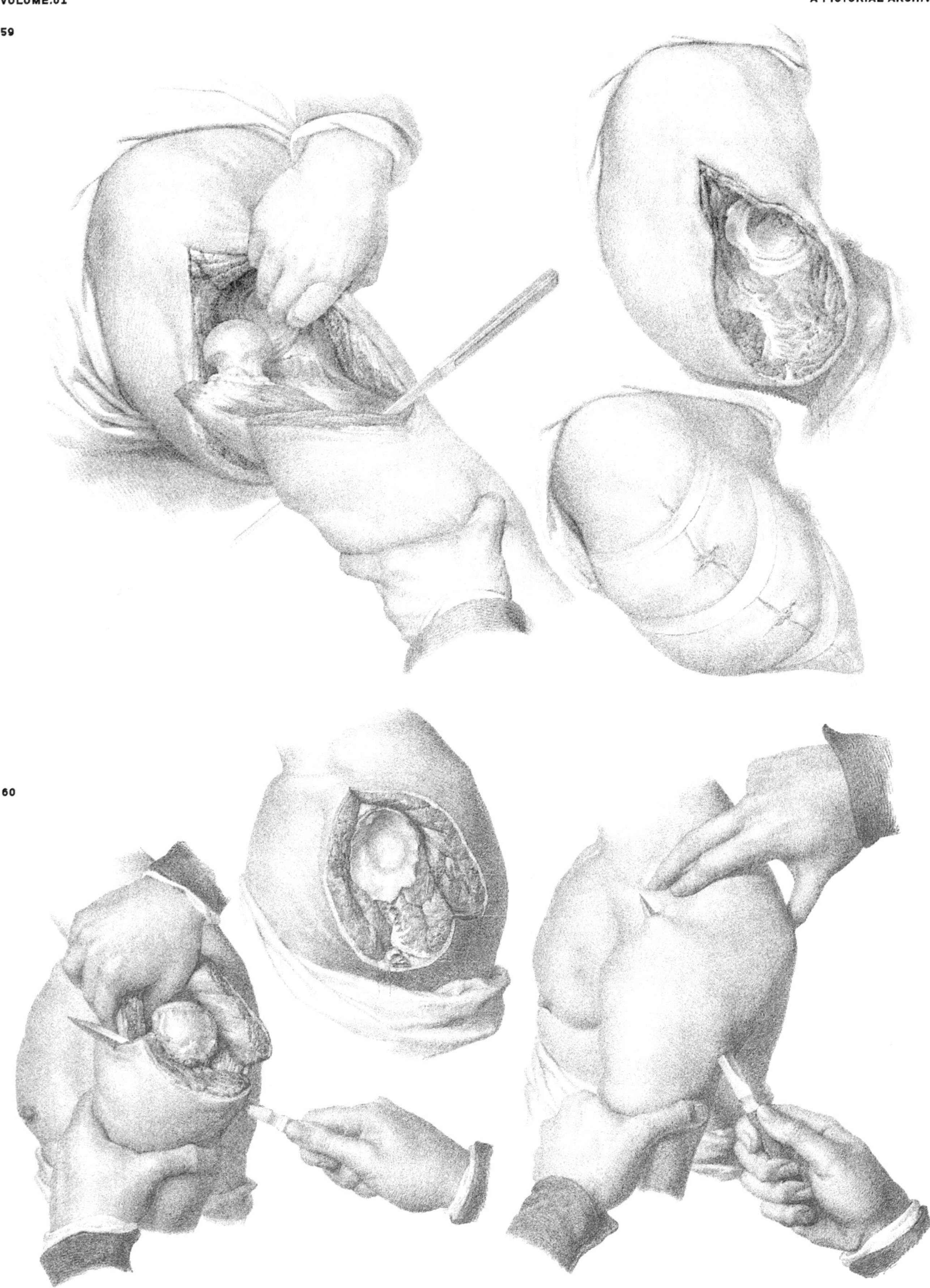

59: Amputation of the leg at the hip and a stump    60: Amputation of the arm at the shoulder.
closure.

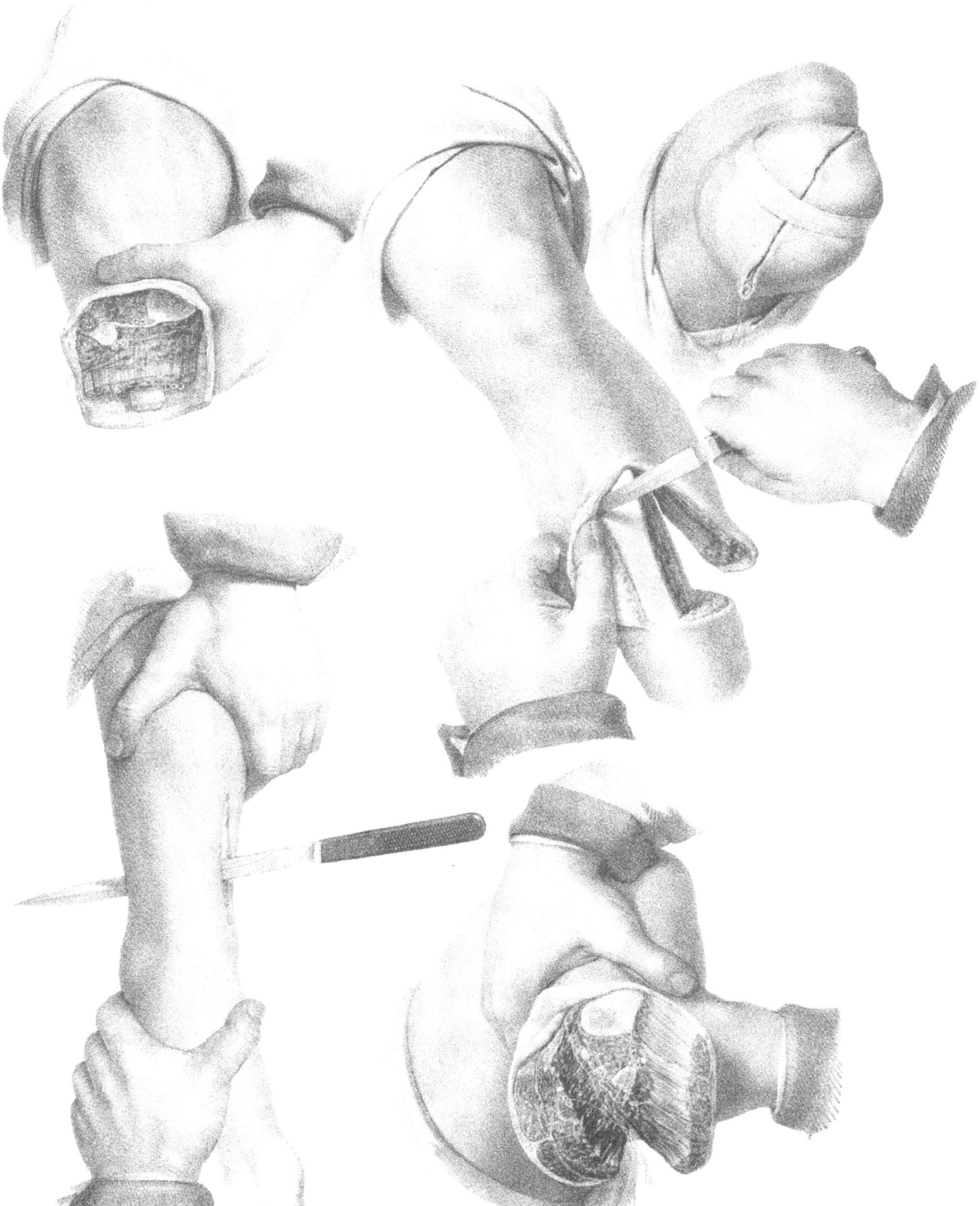

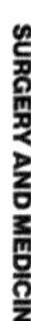

61: Amputation of the lower leg.

62



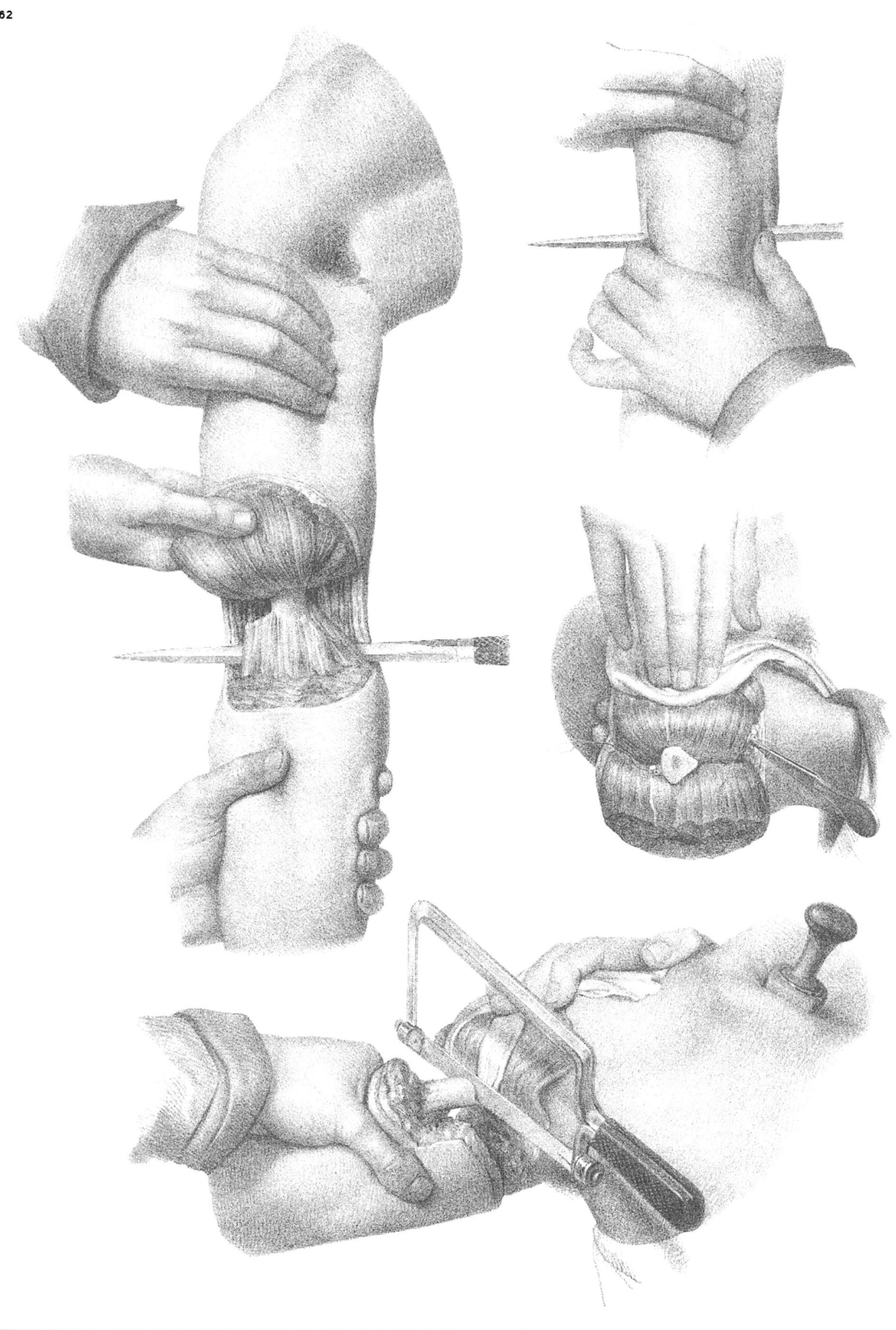

62: Diagrams illustrating the amputation of the
upper and lower arm.

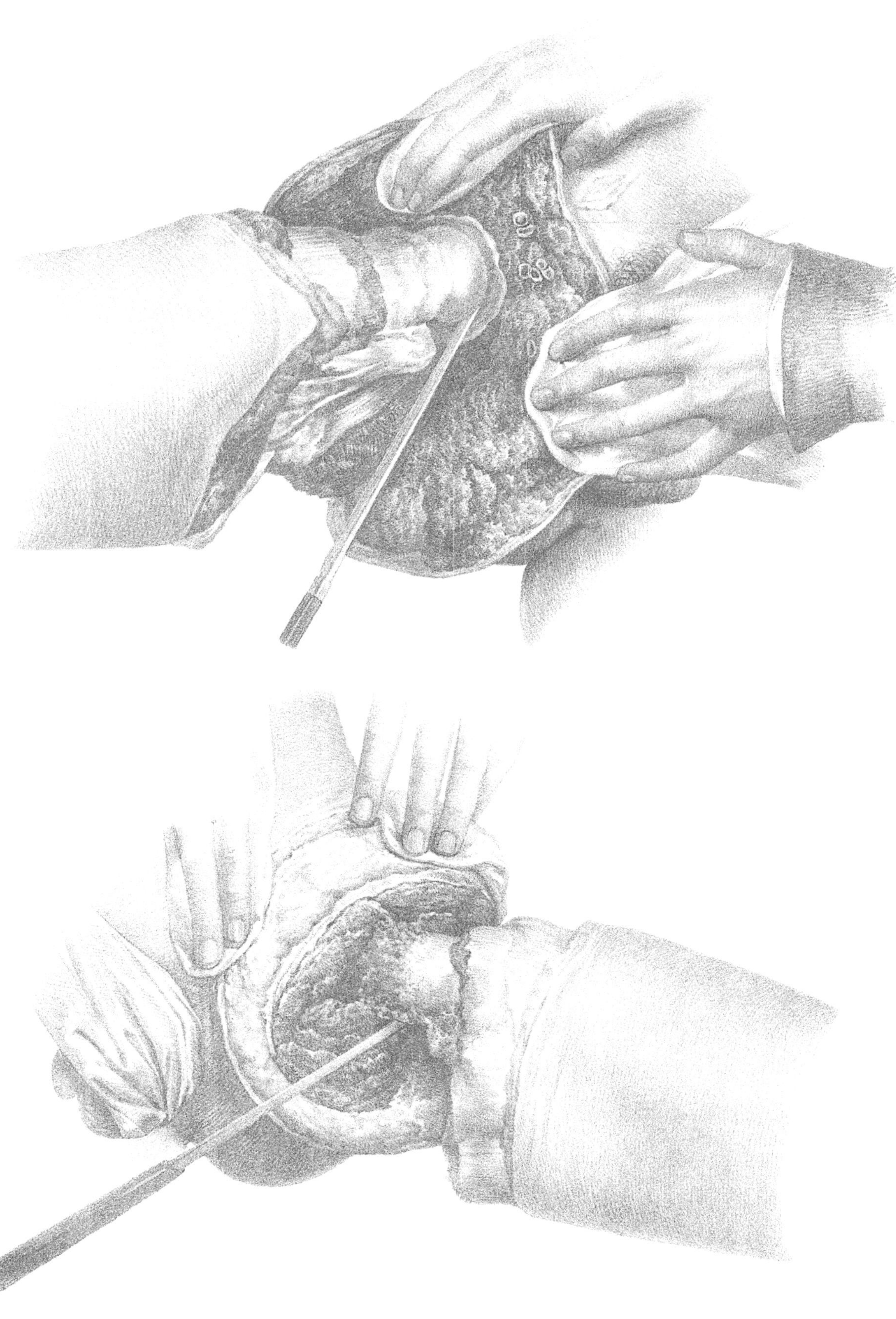

63: Diagrams illustrating the amputation of the
leg at the hip and thigh.

64



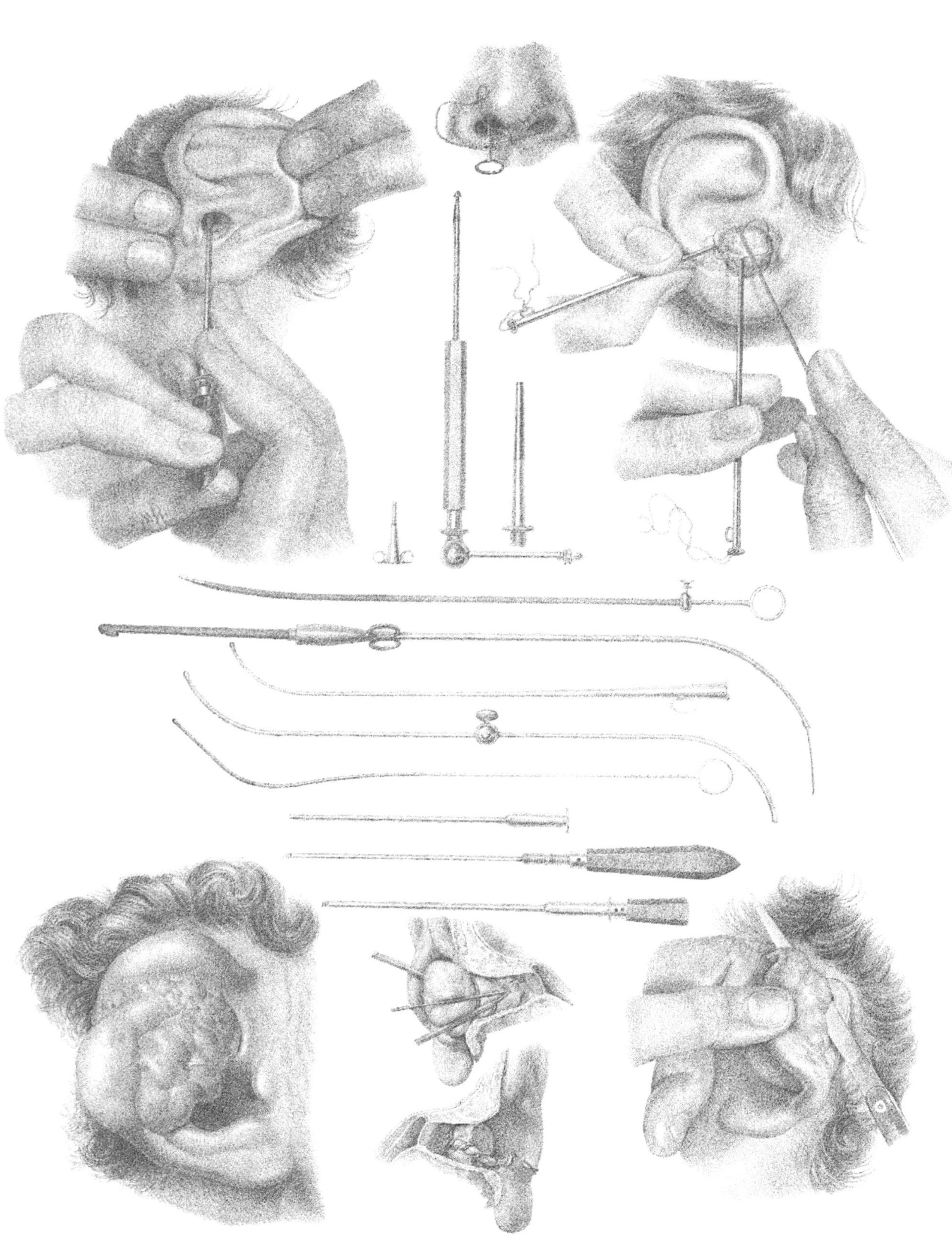

64: Techniques for operating on tumours of
the ear.

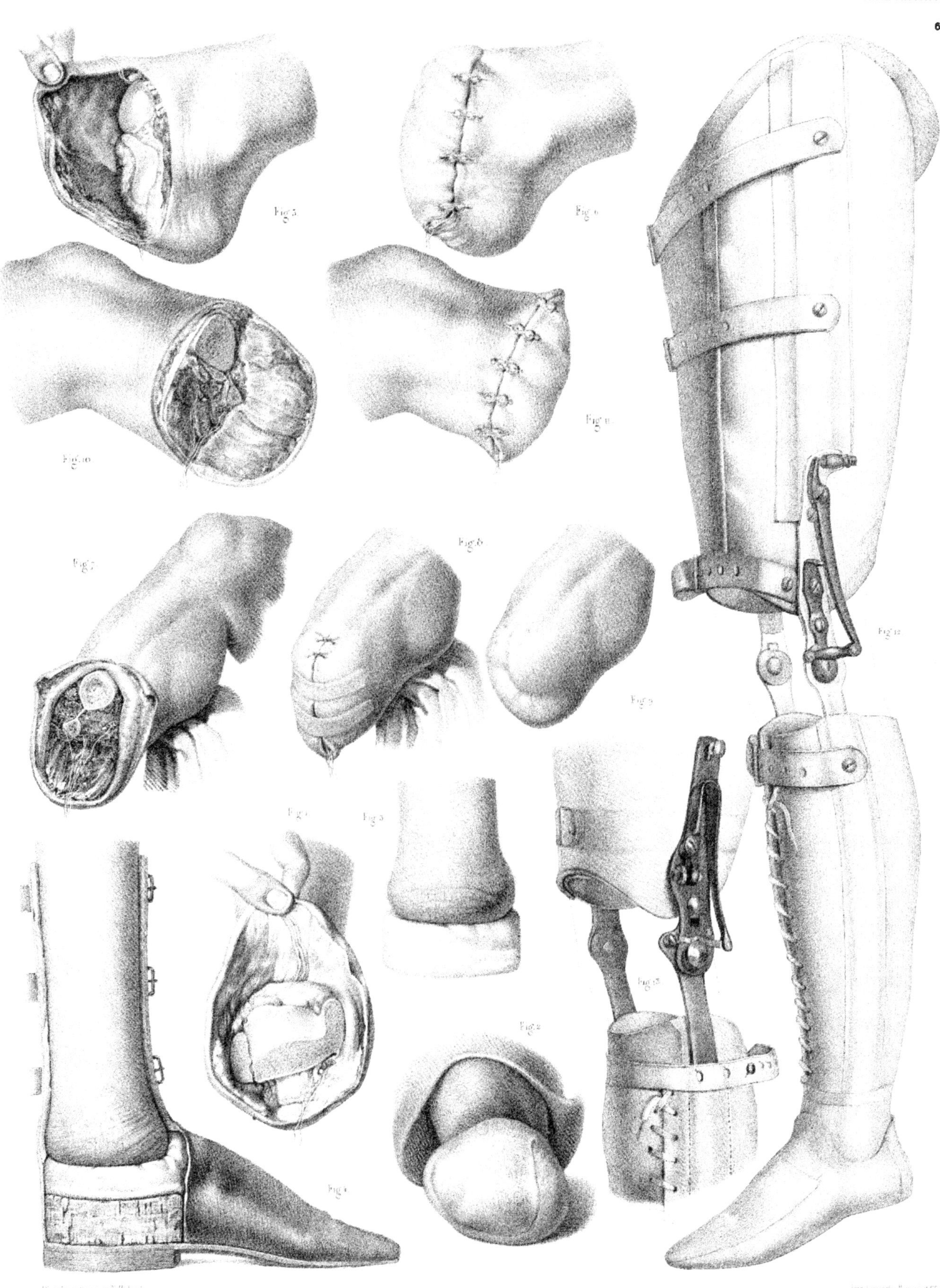

65: Amputation of the leg and prostheses.

66



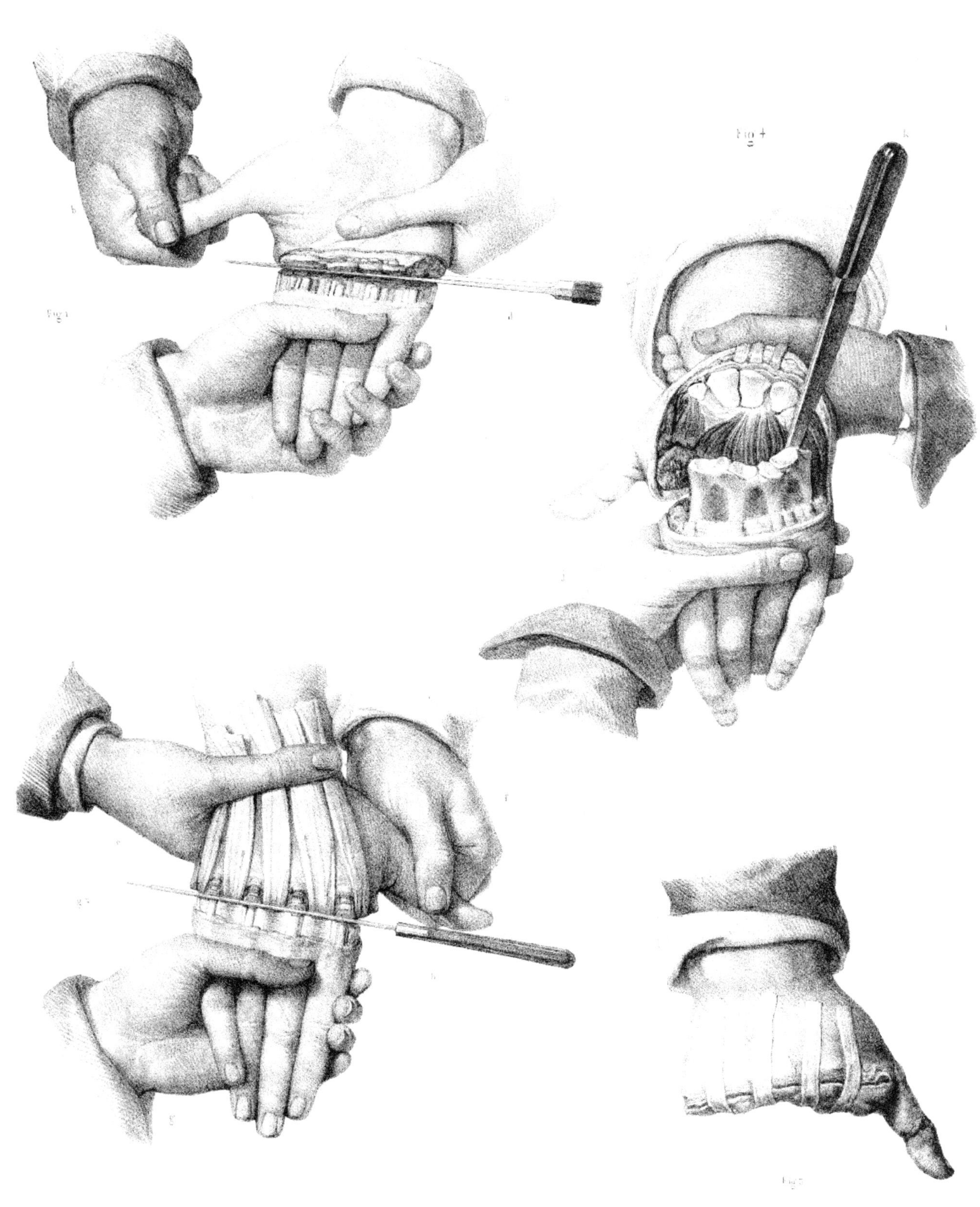

66: Diagrams illustrating the amputation of the
fingers at the metacarpals bones.

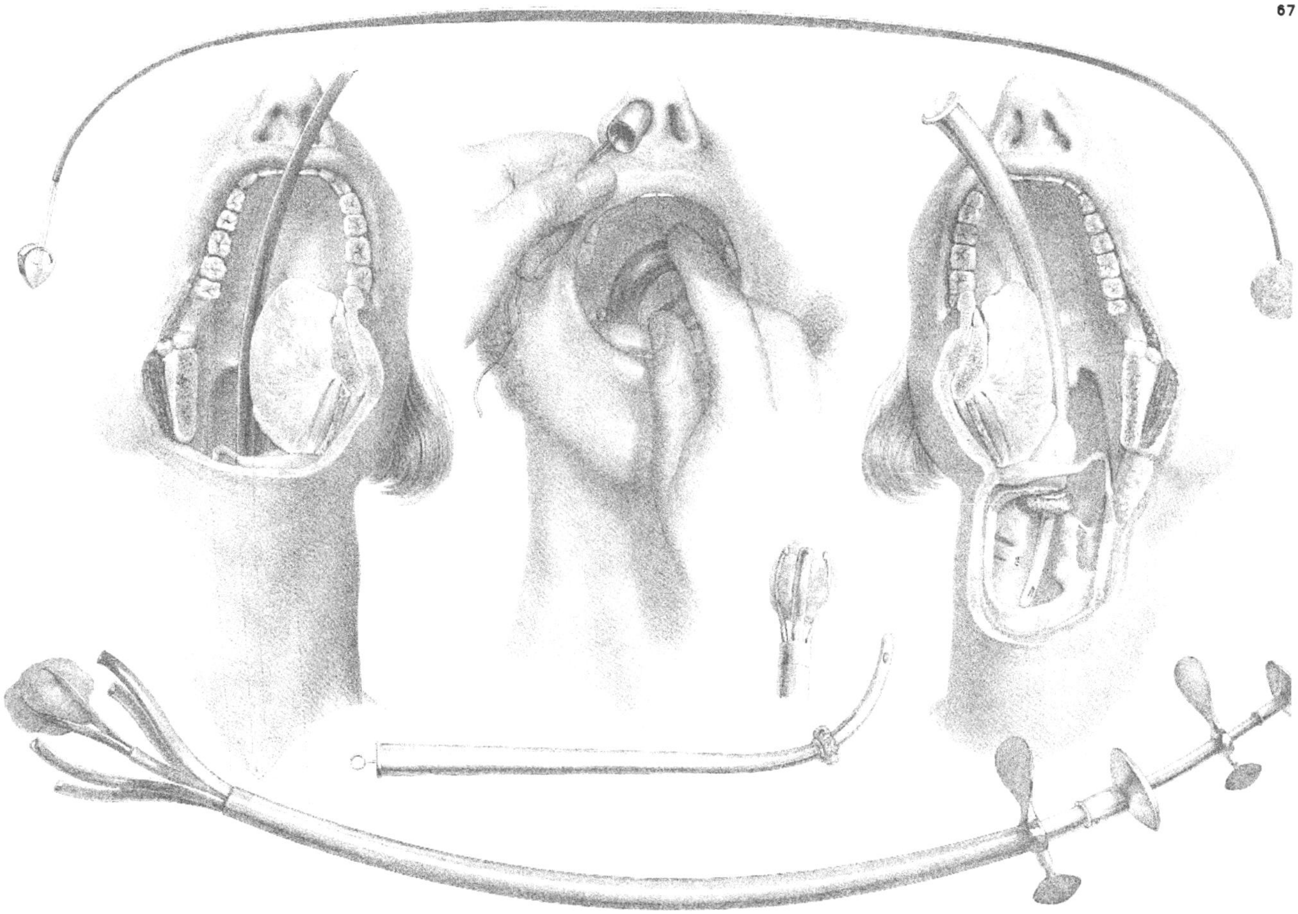

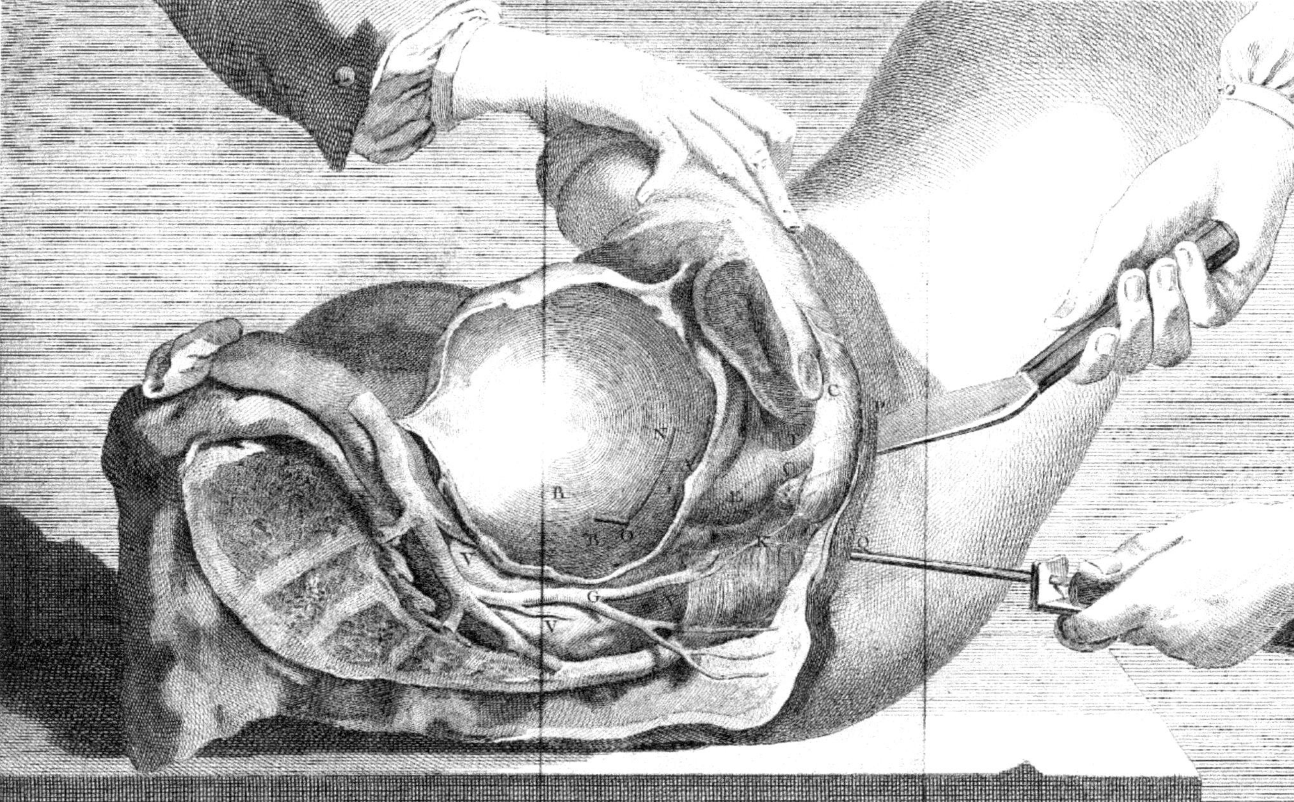



68

67: Instruments for performing surgery on the throat from Traité complet de l'anatomie.

68: Amputation of the leg.

69



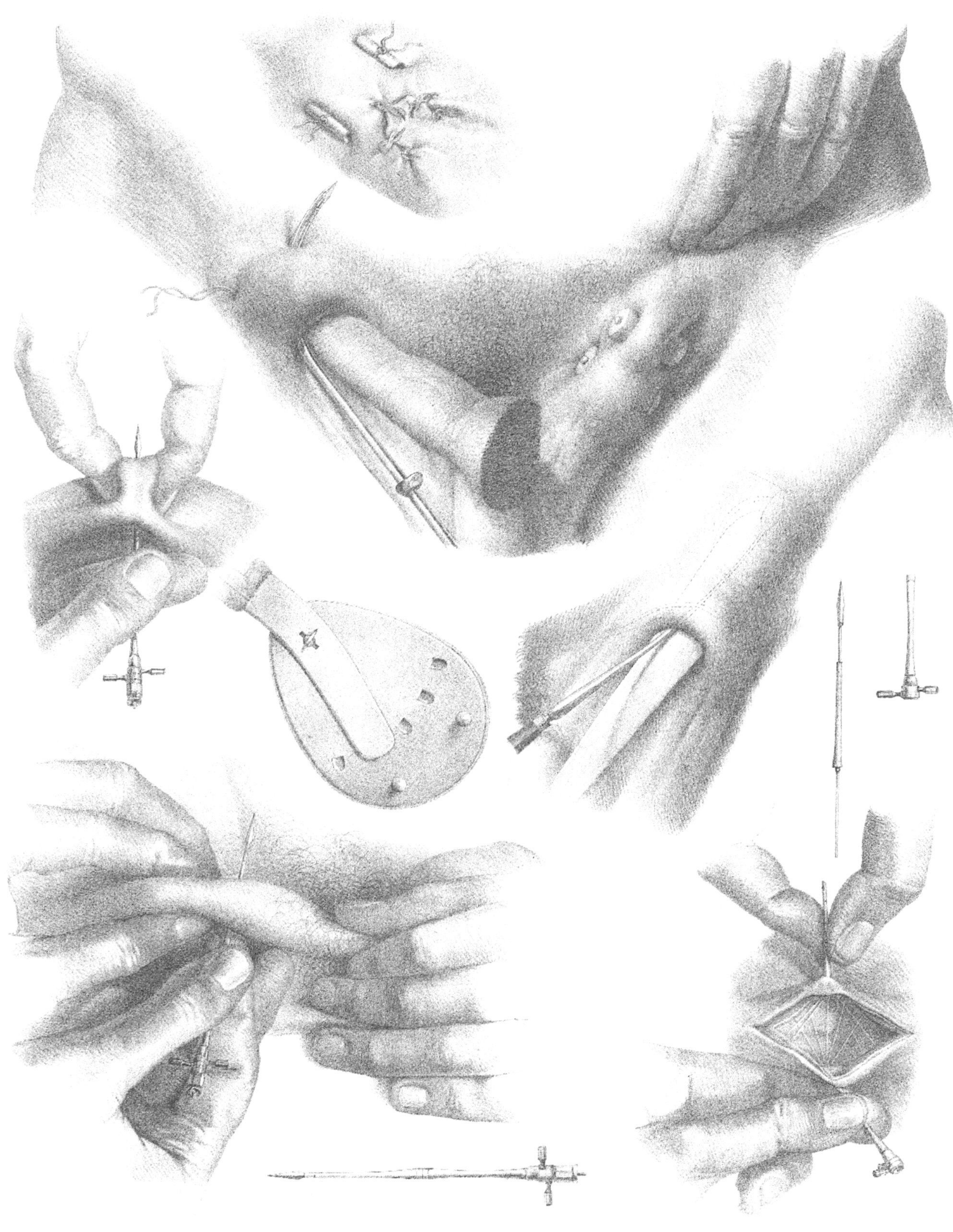

69: Diagram illustrating methods to repair an
inguinal hernia.

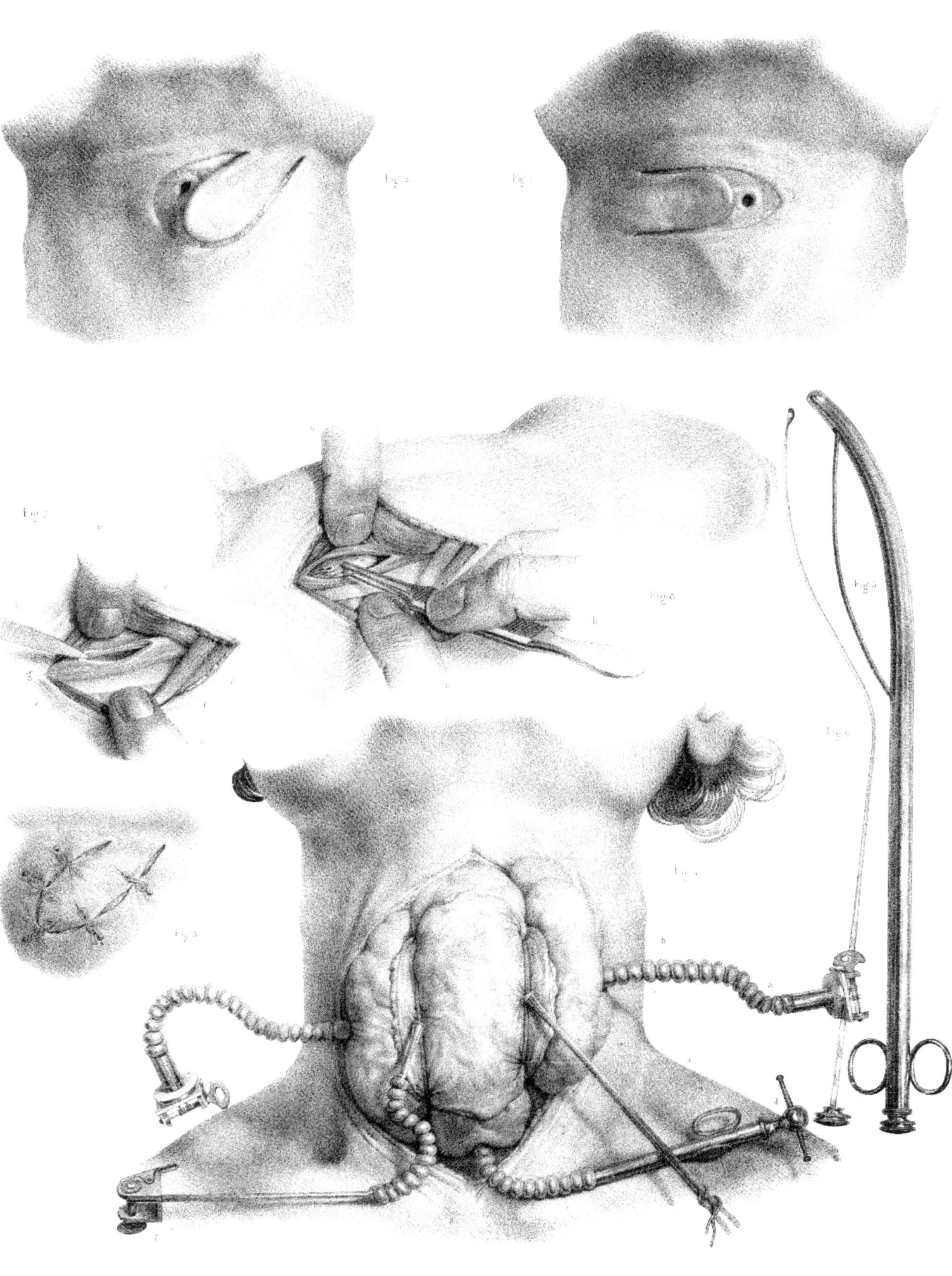



70: Diagram illustrating the surgical procedure of a tracheotomy. Featured in Traité complet de l'anatomie.

71



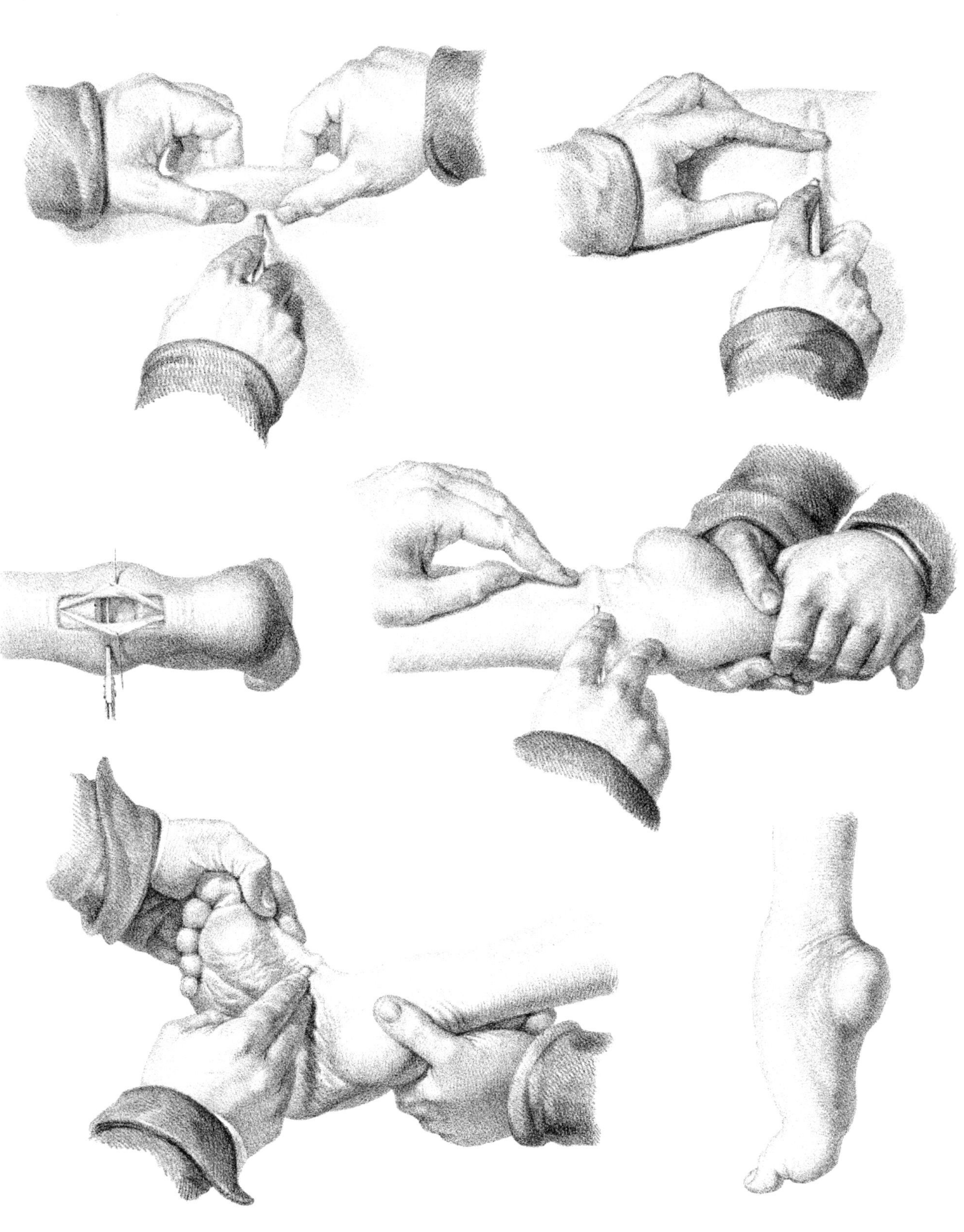

71: Diagram illustrating a surgical technique to correct club foot.

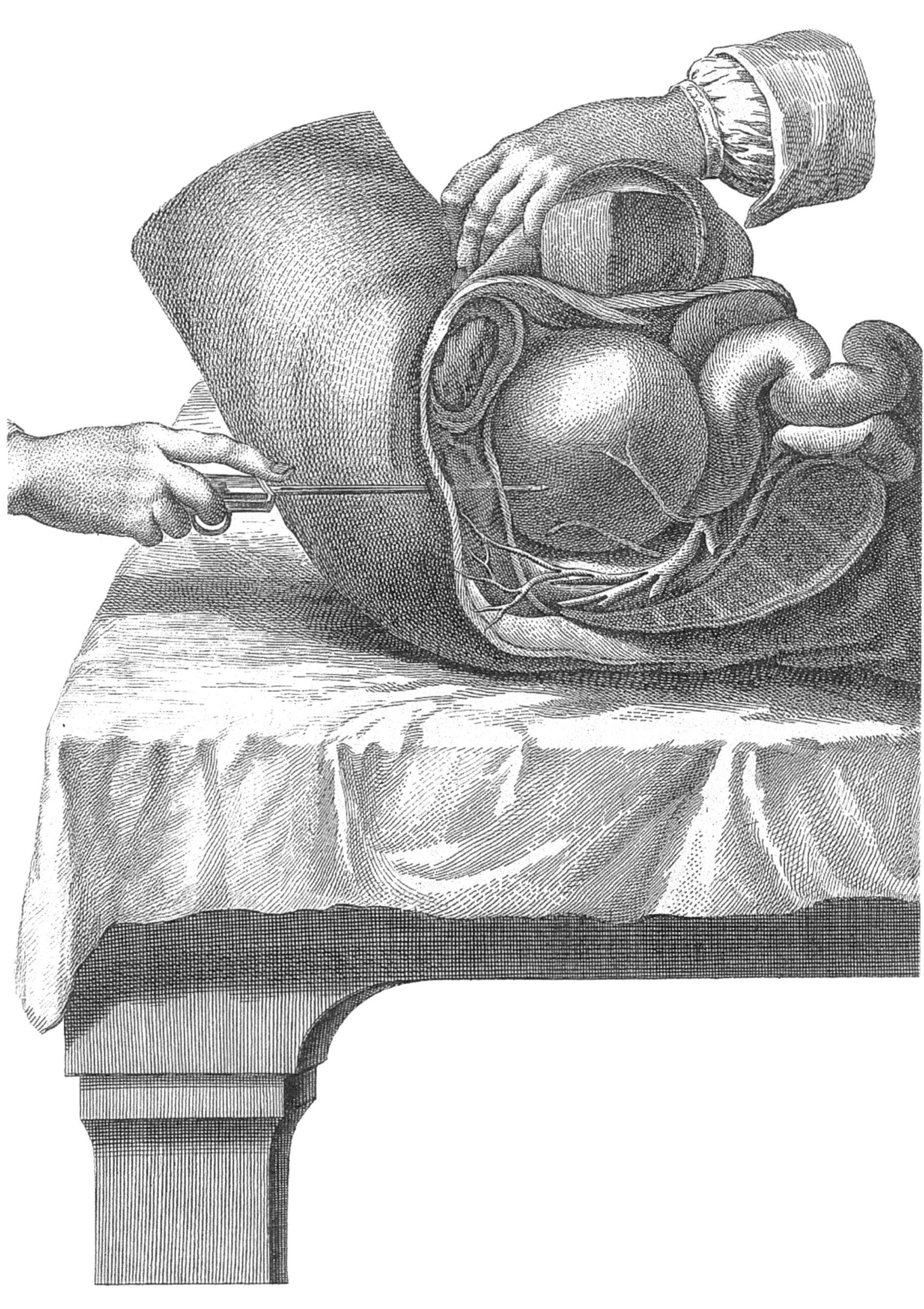

72: A dissection showing the lateral section of
the hypogastrum.

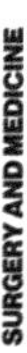

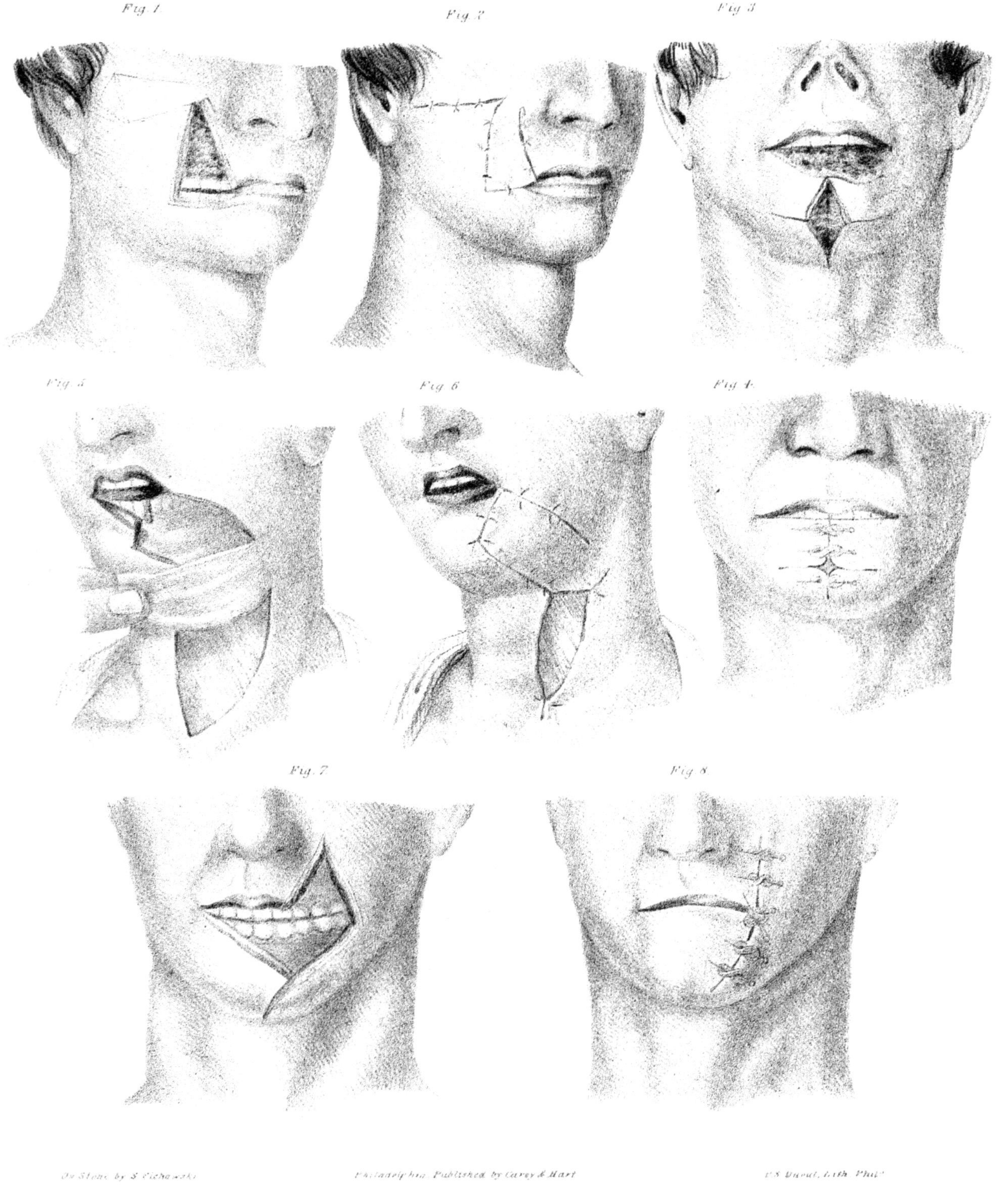

73: Illustration of operative surgery

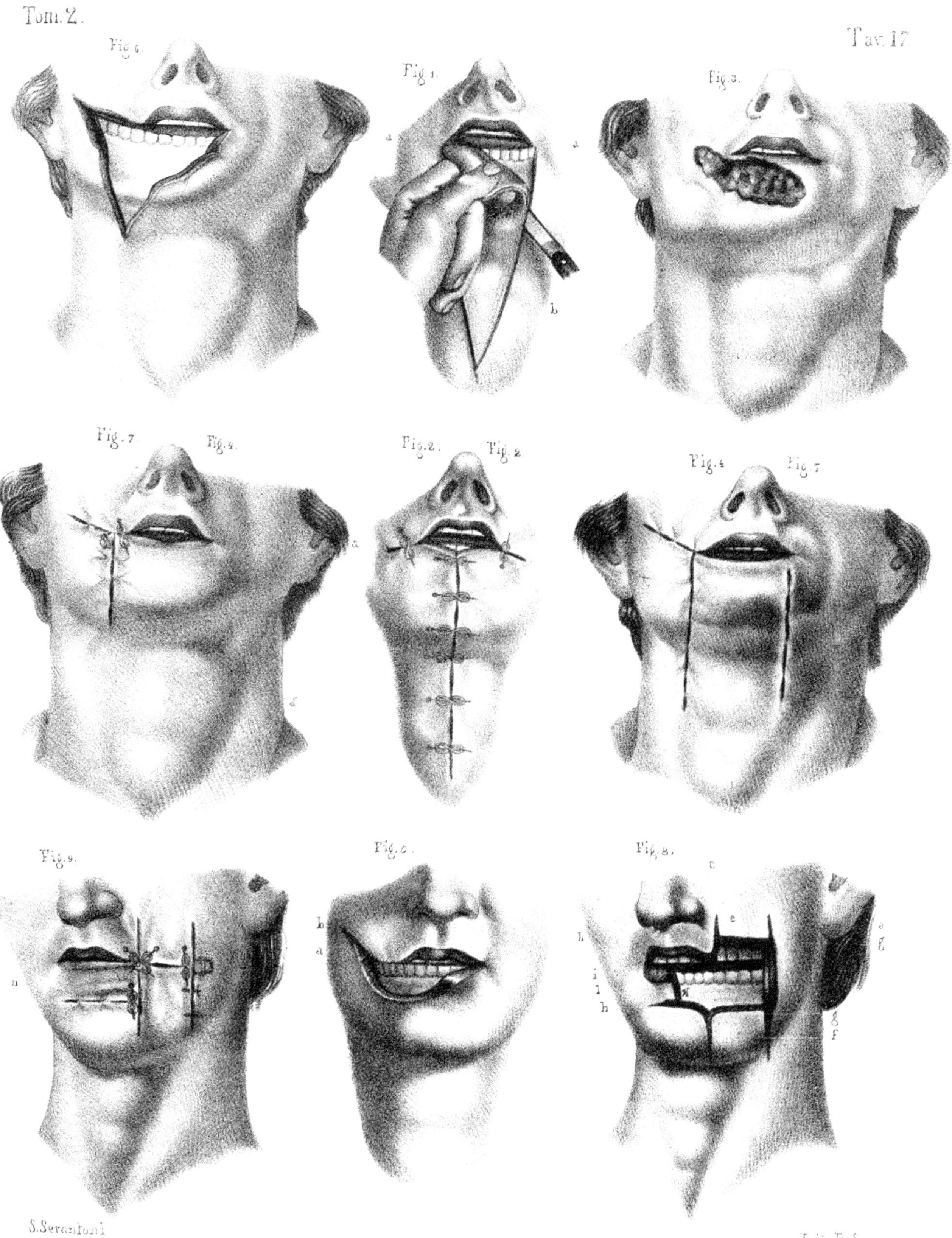
Tom. 2.
Tav. 17.
Fig. 6.
Fig. 1.
Fig. 3.
Fig. 7.
Fig. 4.
Fig. 2.
Fig. 3.
Fig. 4.
Fig. 7.
Fig. 9.
Fig. 6.
Fig. 8.
S. Seranfoni
SURGERY AND MEDICINE

75



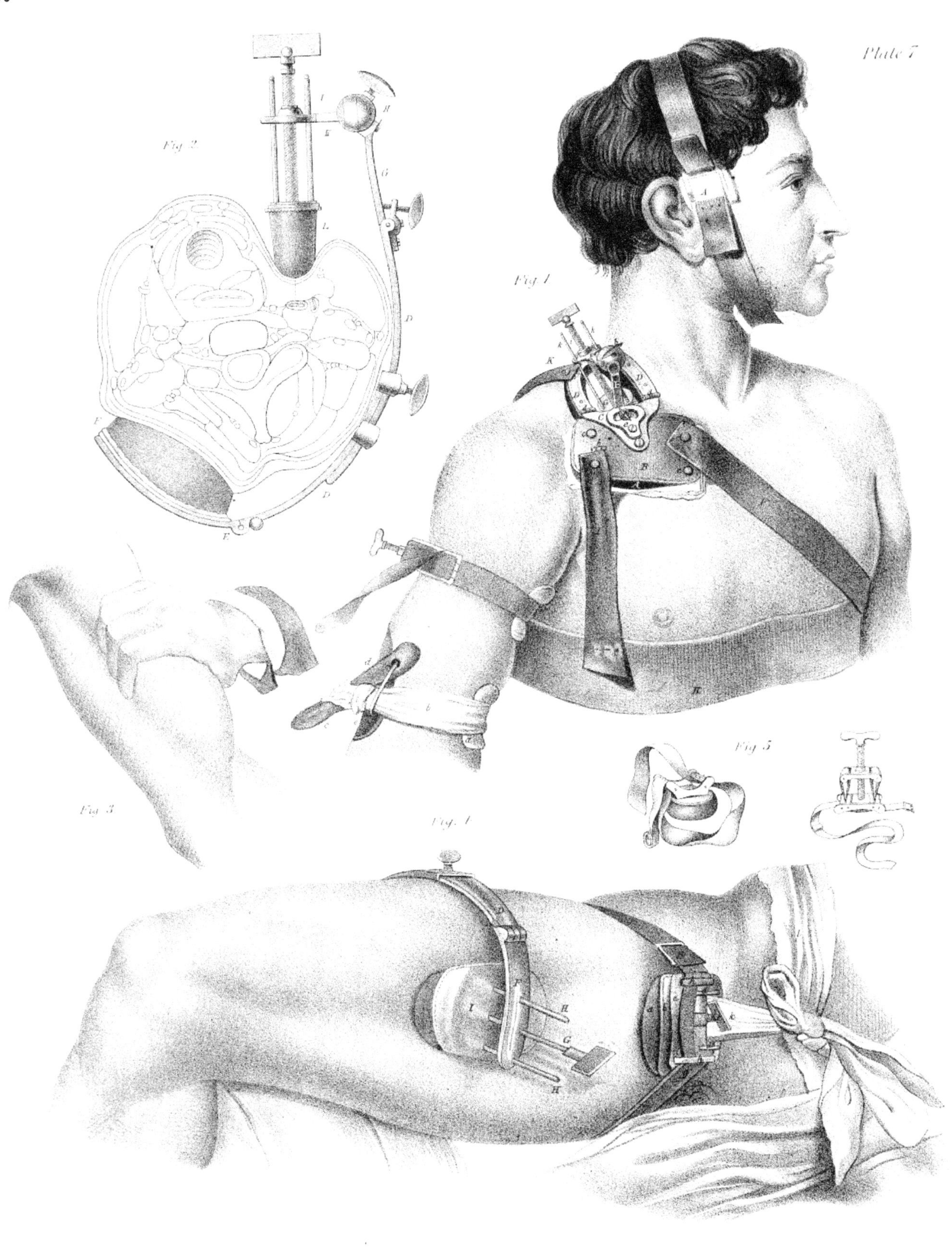


75: A diagram illustrating the compression of
the arteries.

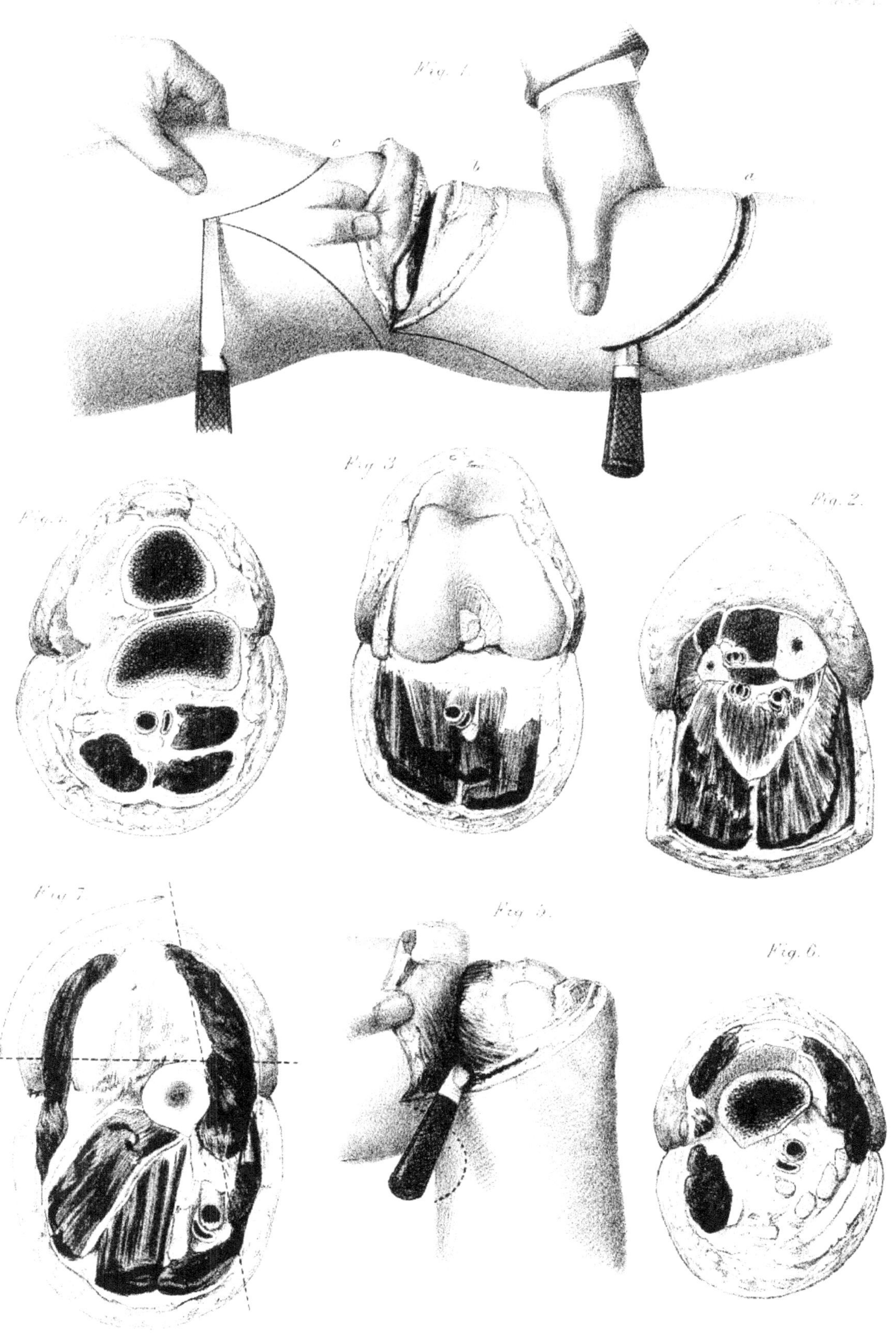


76: A diagram illustrating the amputation of the
leg, knee, and thigh.

77



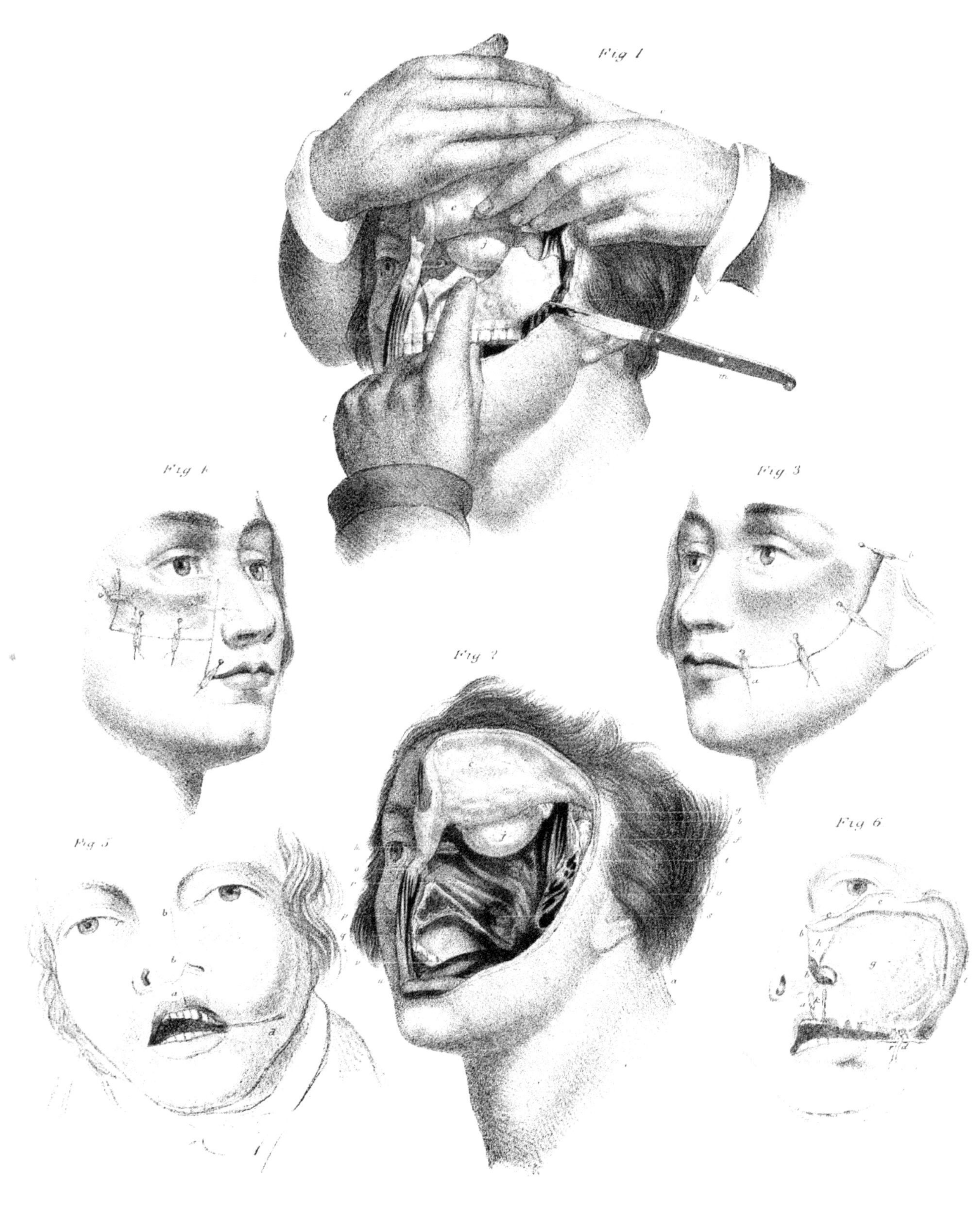


77: Diagram illustrating a resection of the upper jaw.

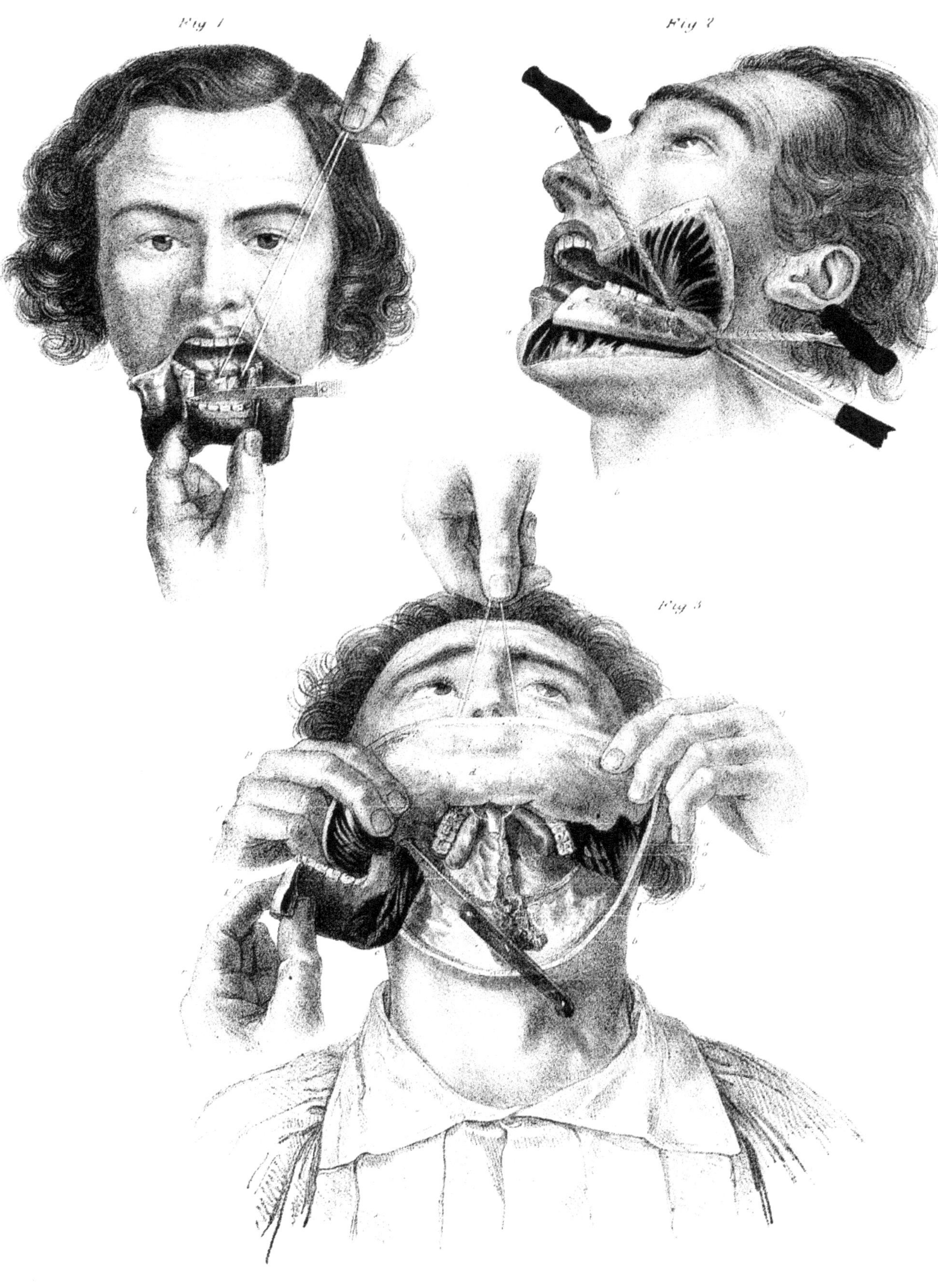




78: Diagram illustrating a resection of the
lower jaw.

79



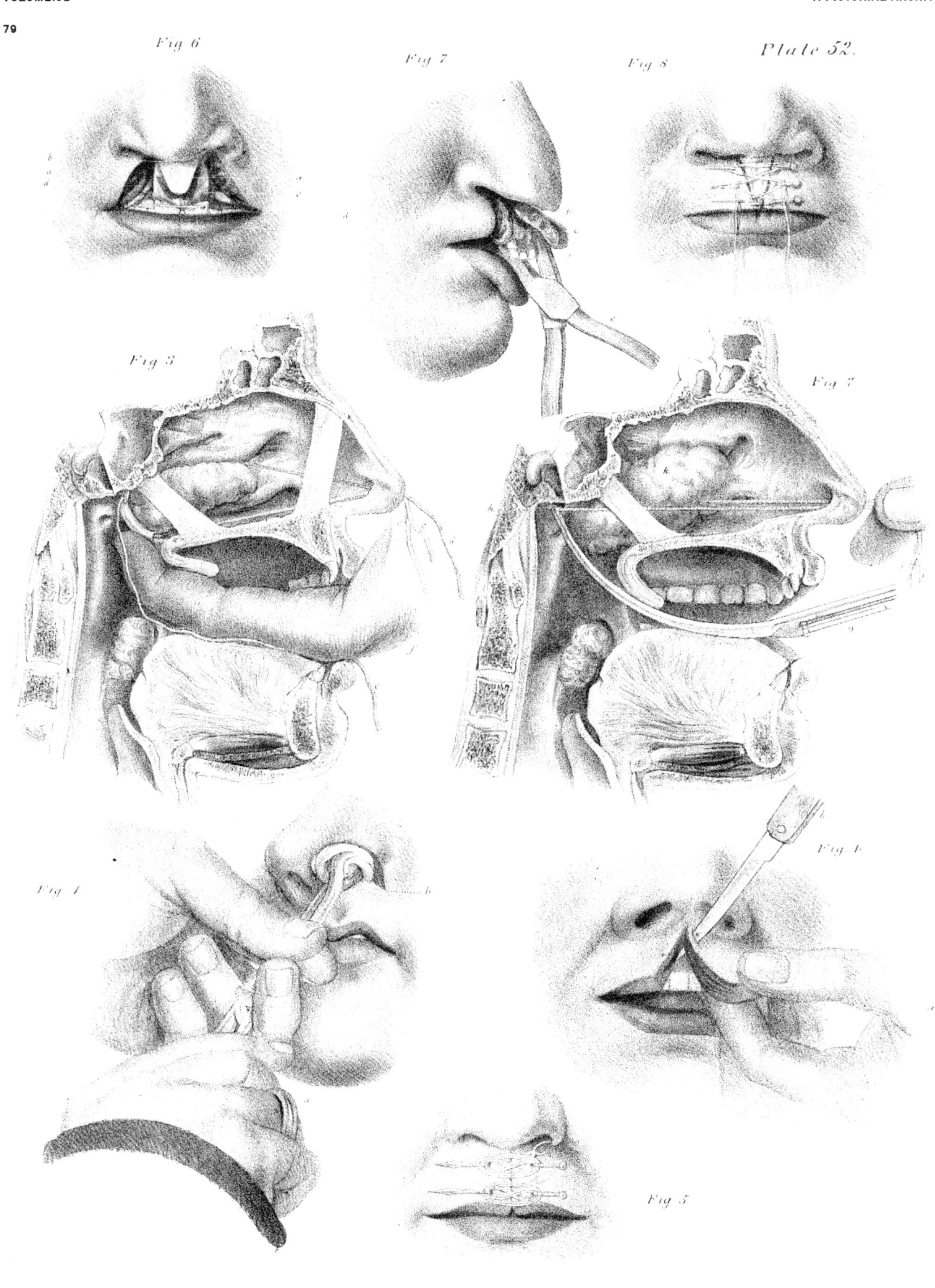


79: Diagram illustrating surgical techniques for
nasal polypi and hare-lip.

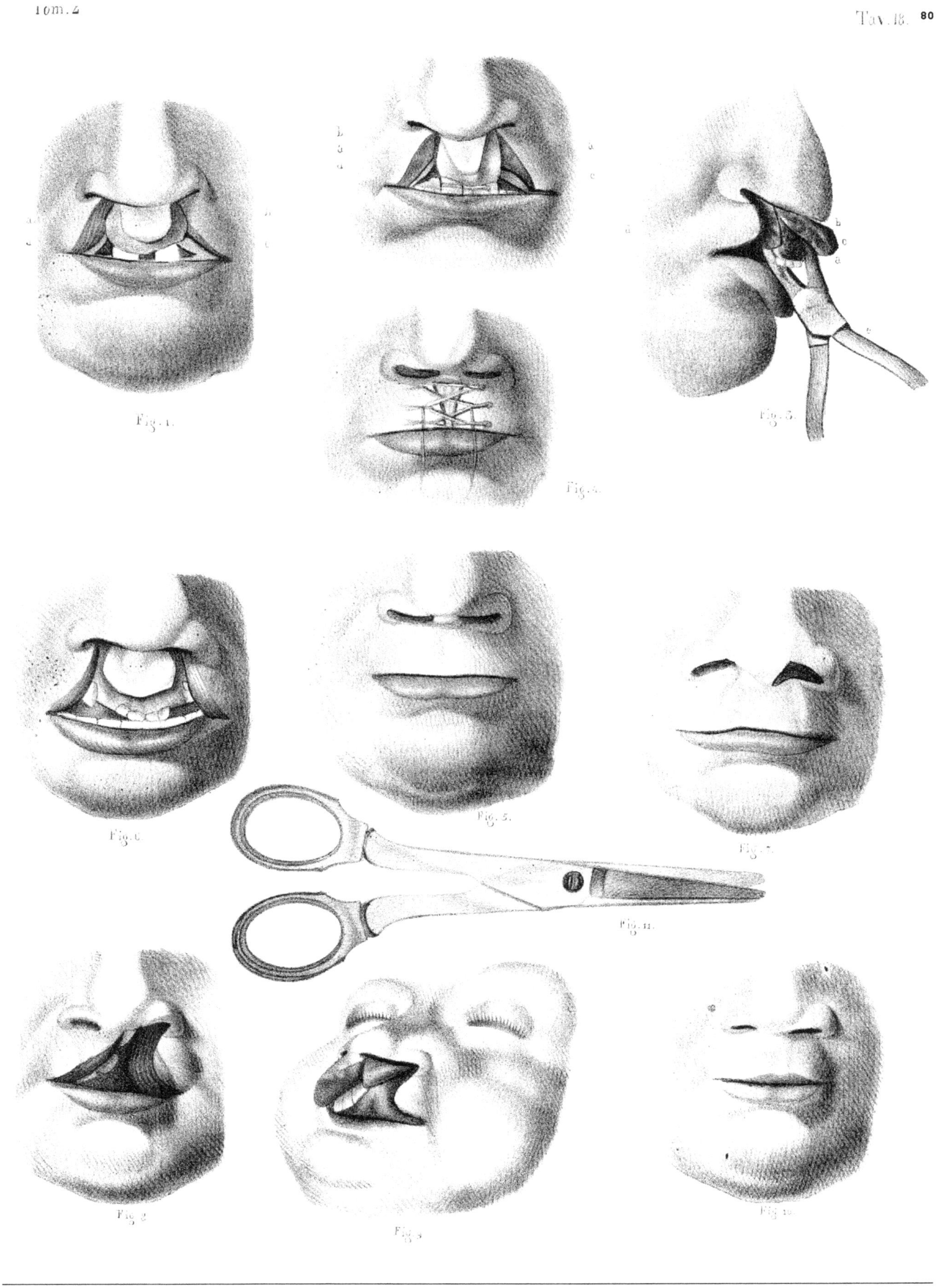

80: Diagram illustrating surgery to repair a cleft lip.

81

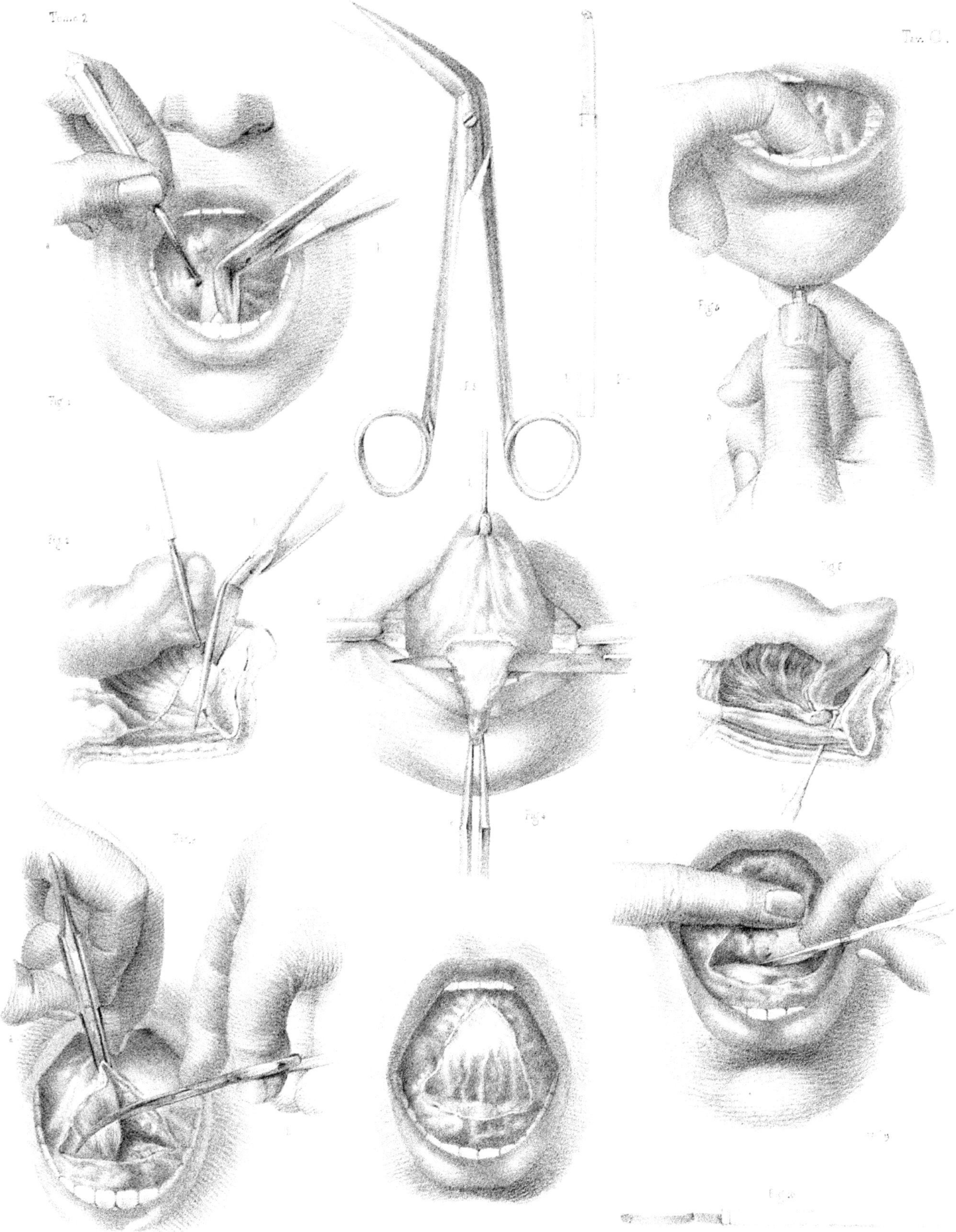

81: Surgical methods being performed on the tongue.

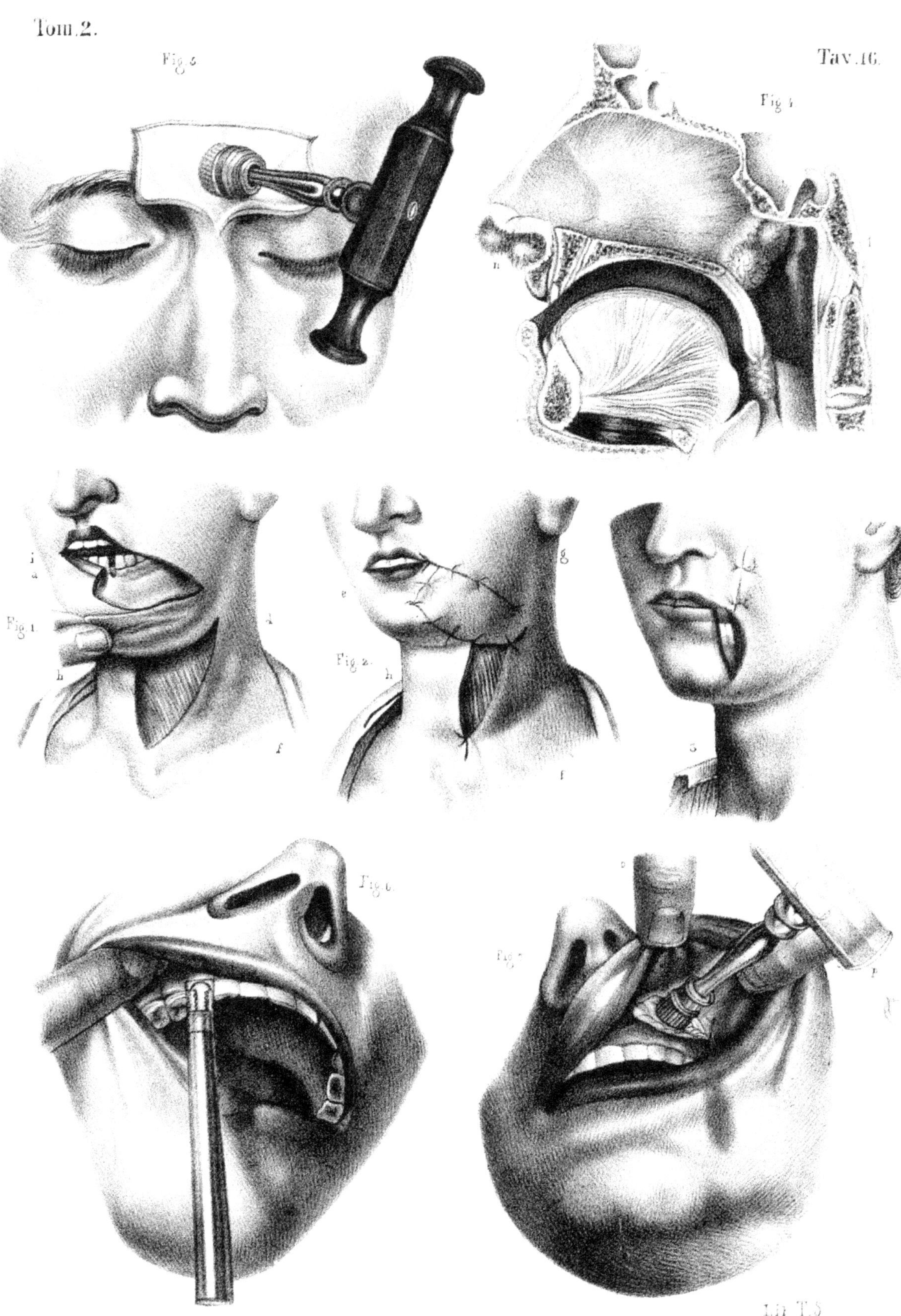




82: Operative techniques featured in Iconografia
d'anatomia.

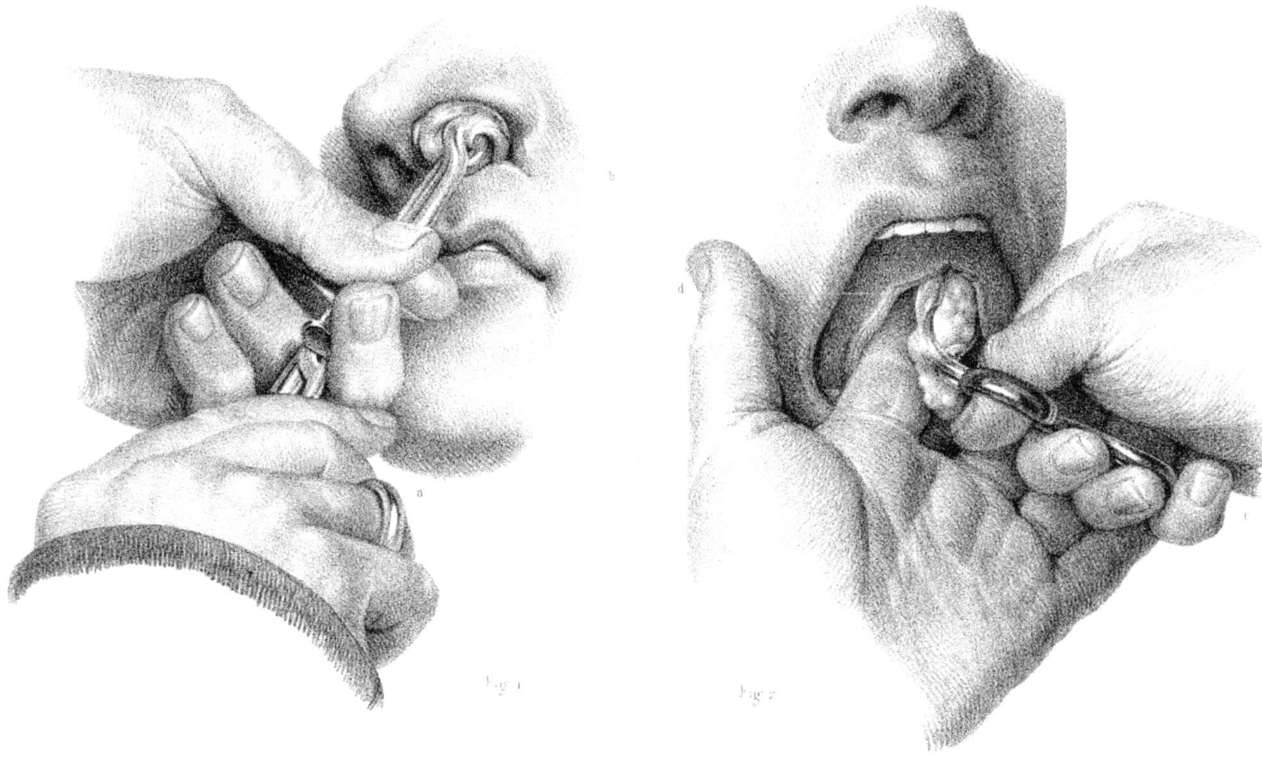

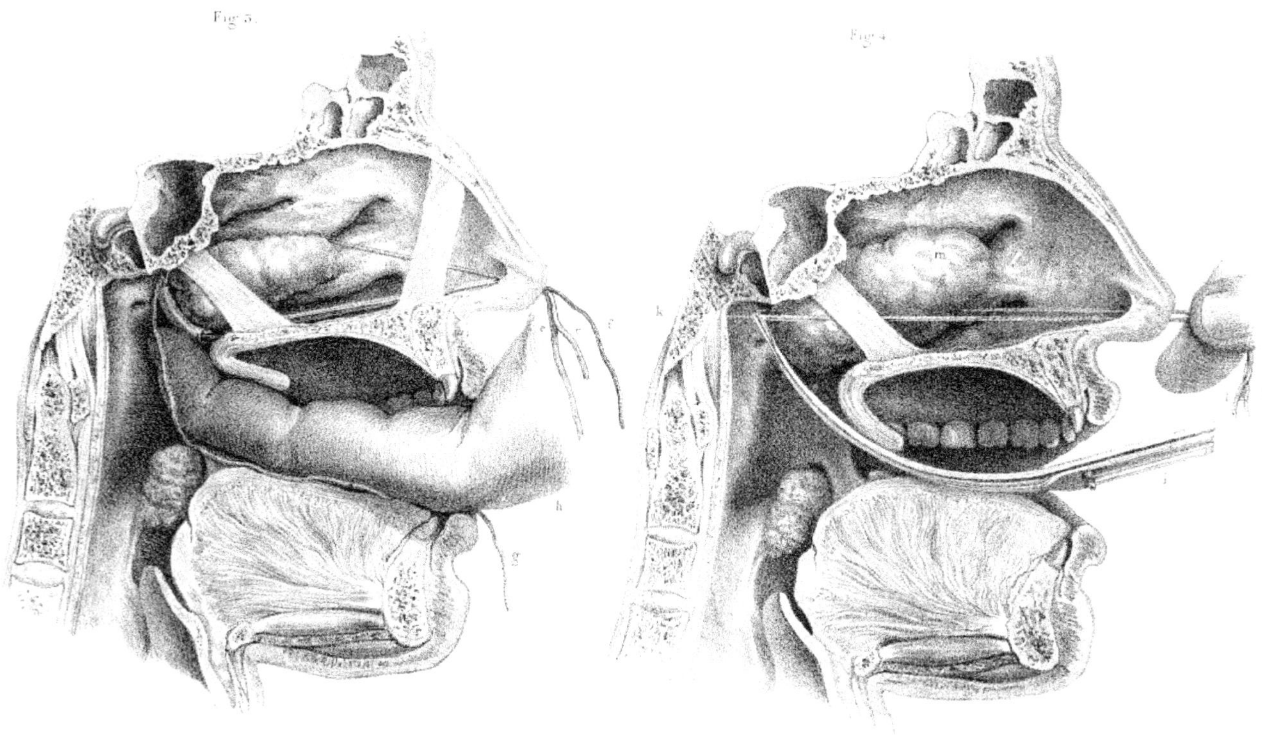

83: Diagram illustrating techniques for operating
on nasal polyps.

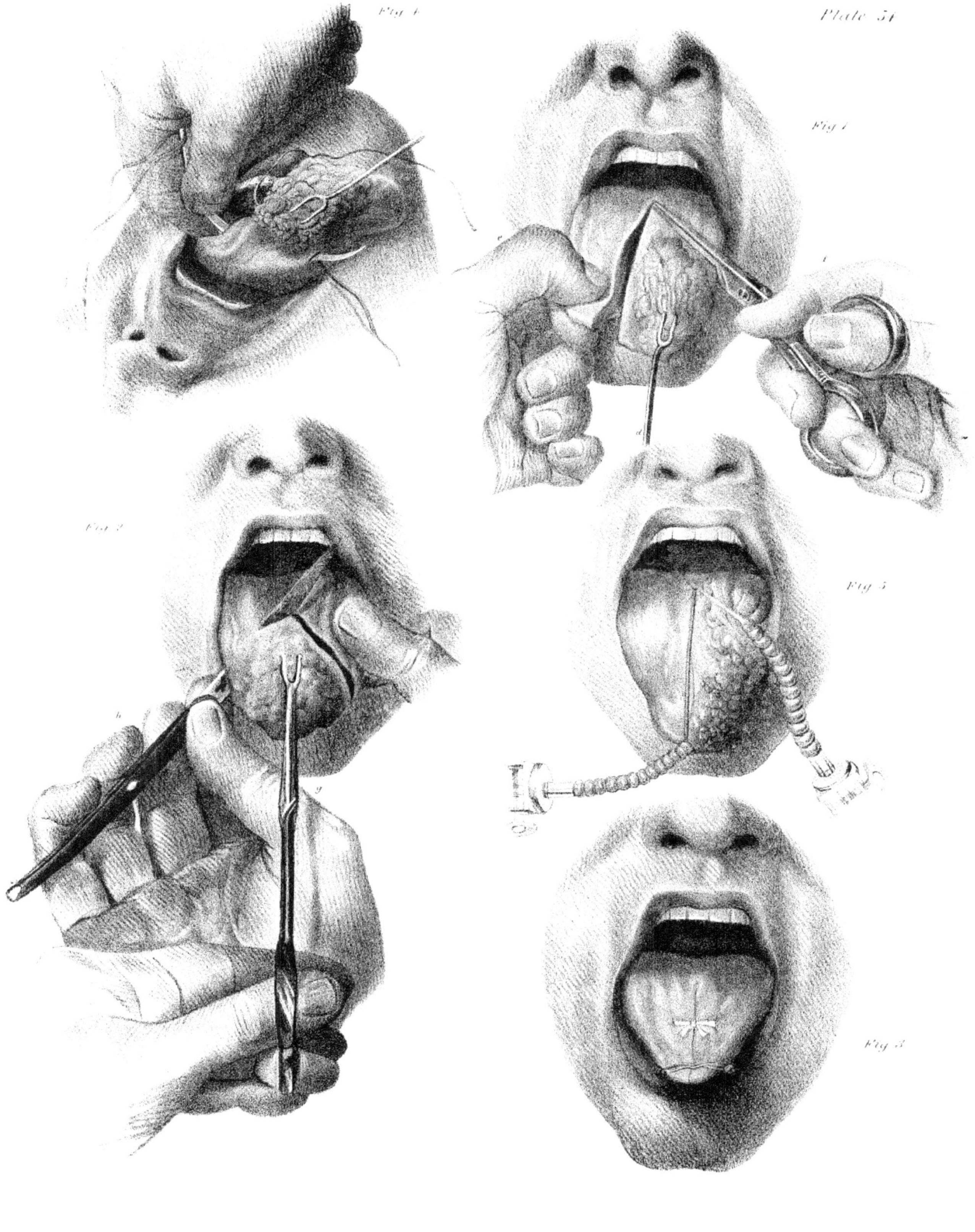

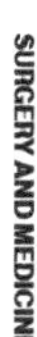


84: Diagram illustrating surgery for cancer of
the tongue.

85



Fig. 1.

Fig. 2.

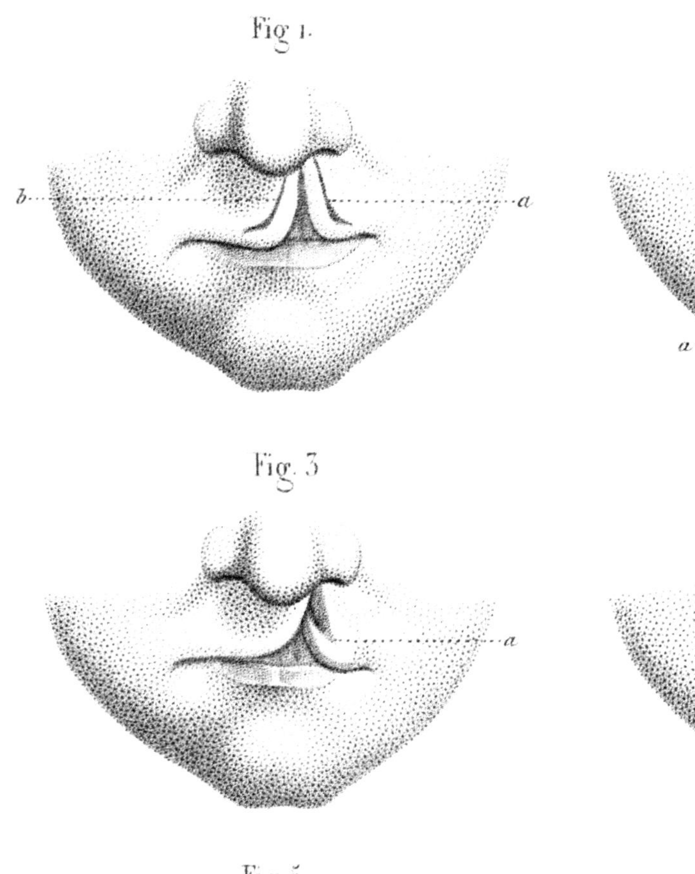
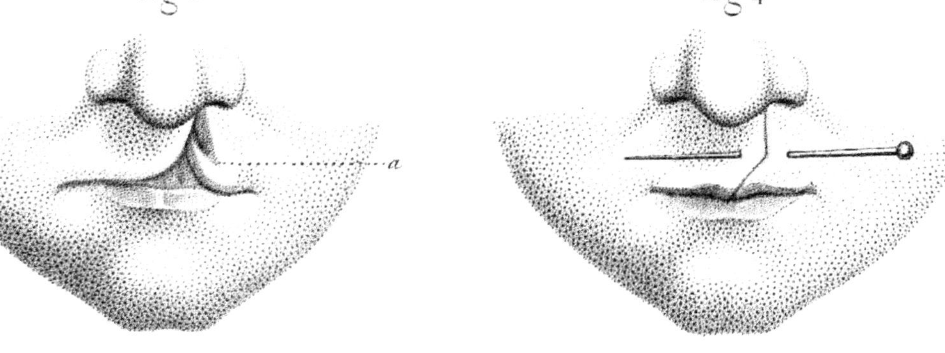


Fig. 3.

Fig. 4.



Fig. 5.

Fig. 6.

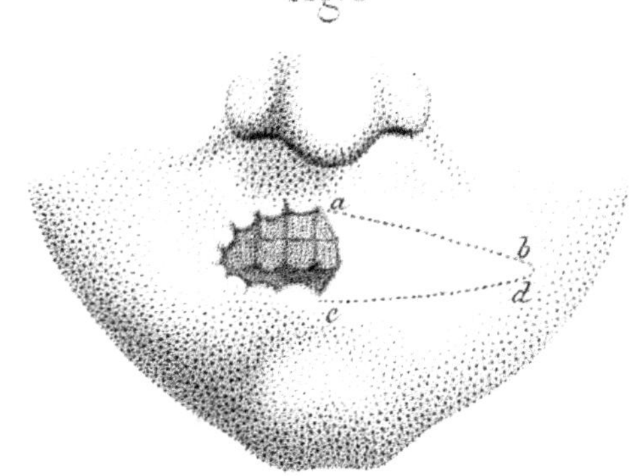
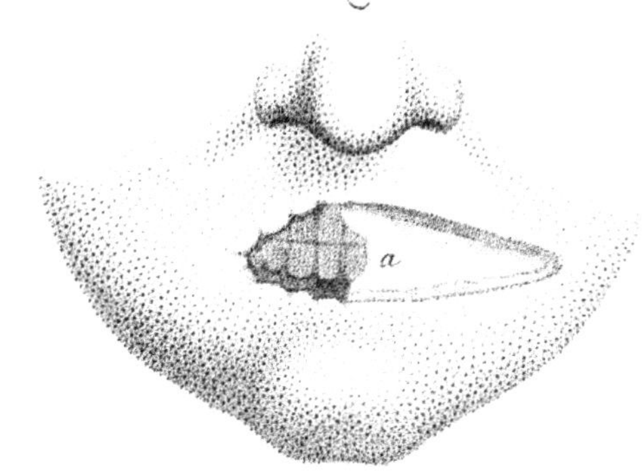


Fig. 7.

Fig. 8.

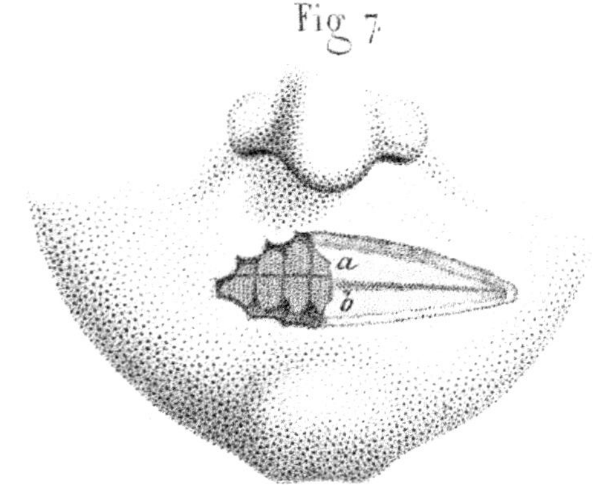
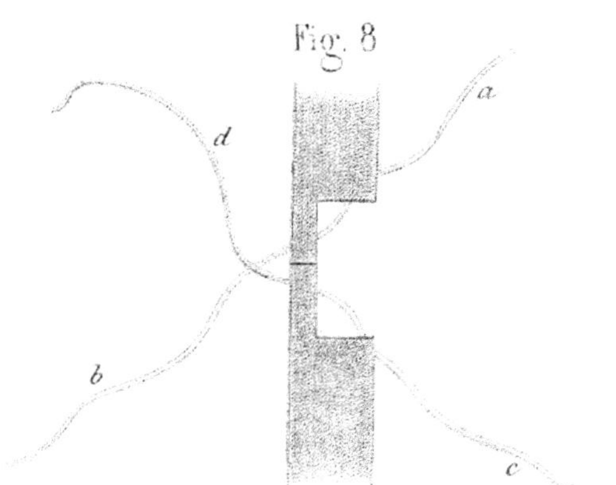

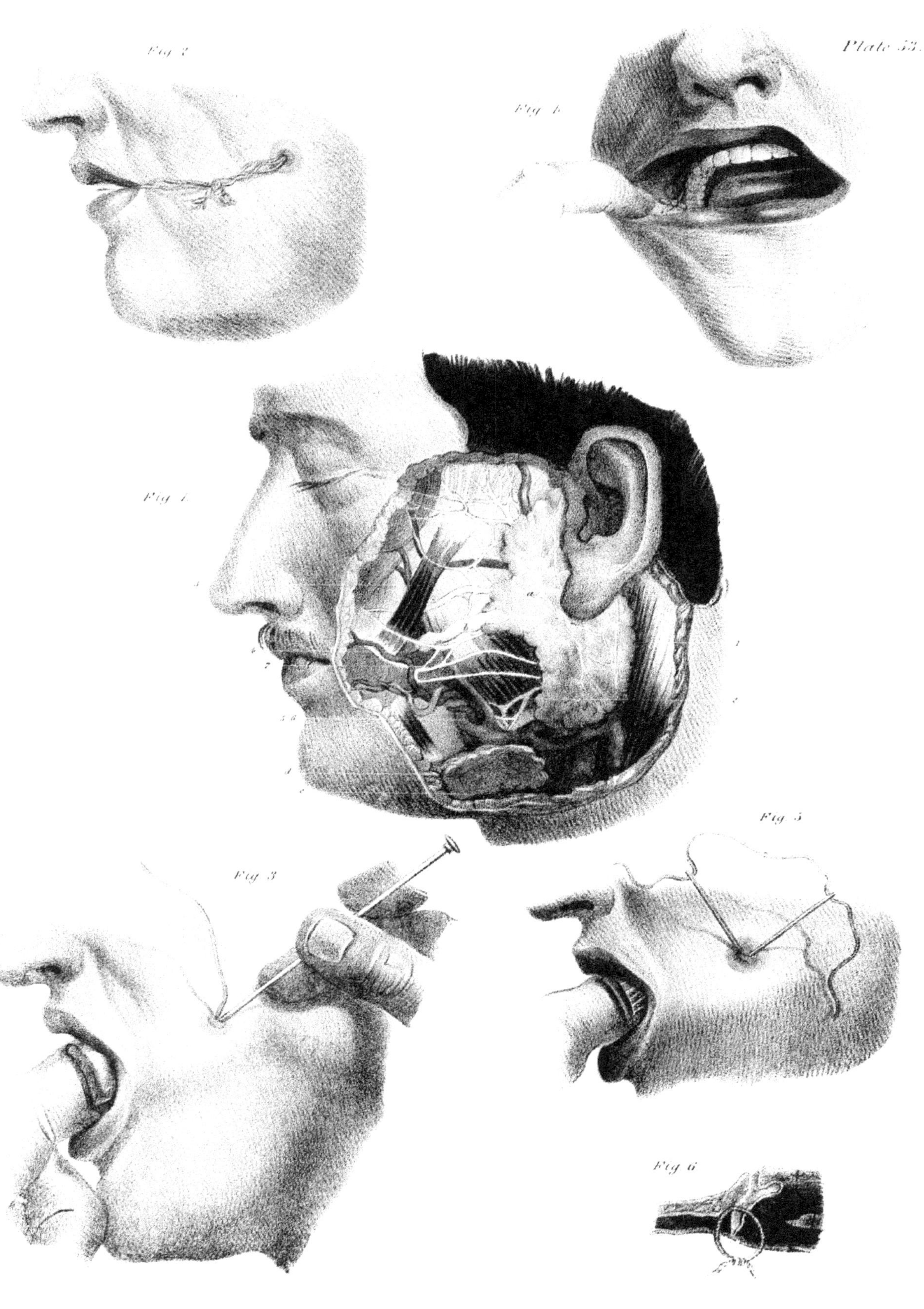




86: Diagram illustrating surgical technique to
remove a salivary fistula.

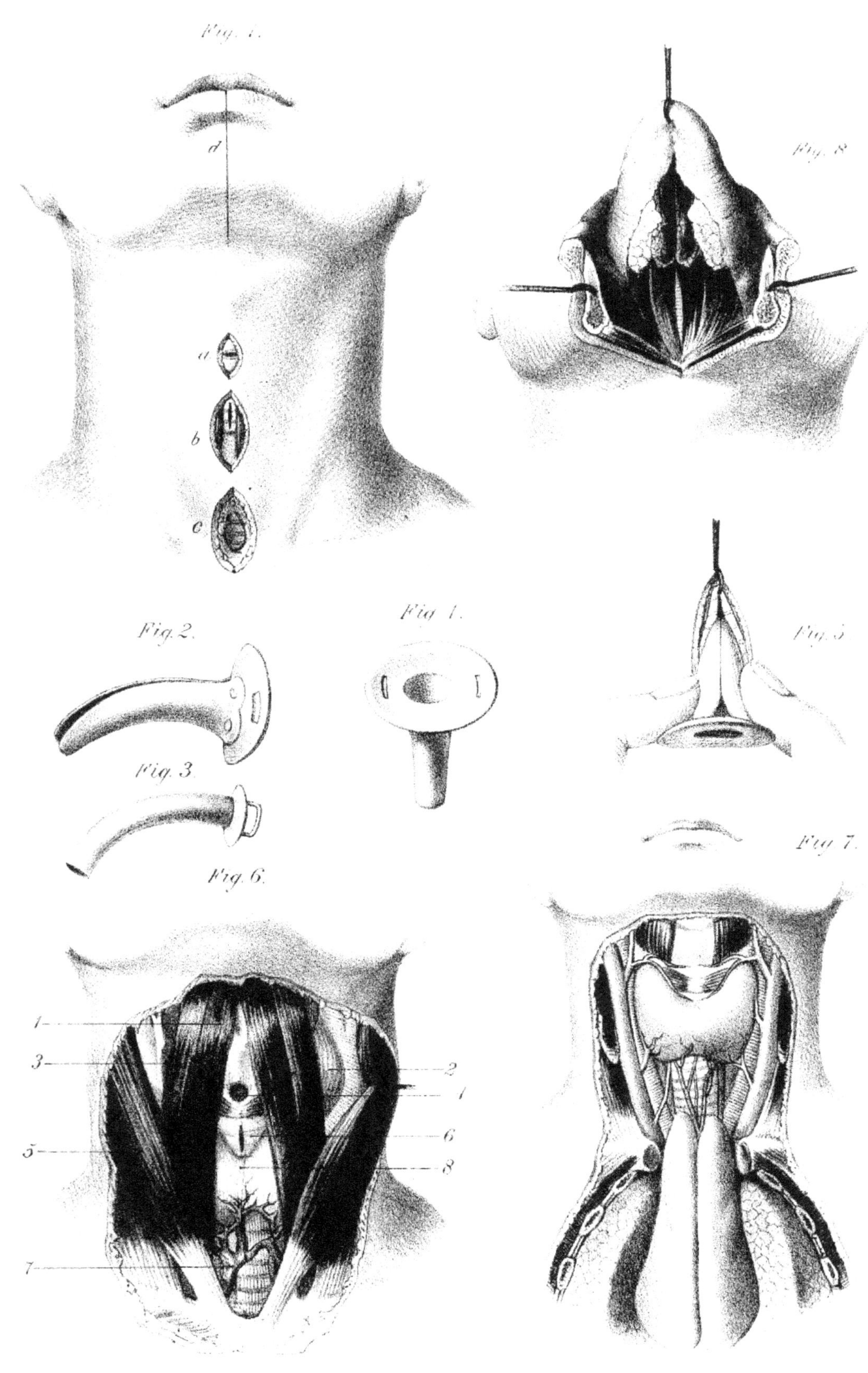


87: Diagram illustrating operative surgery.

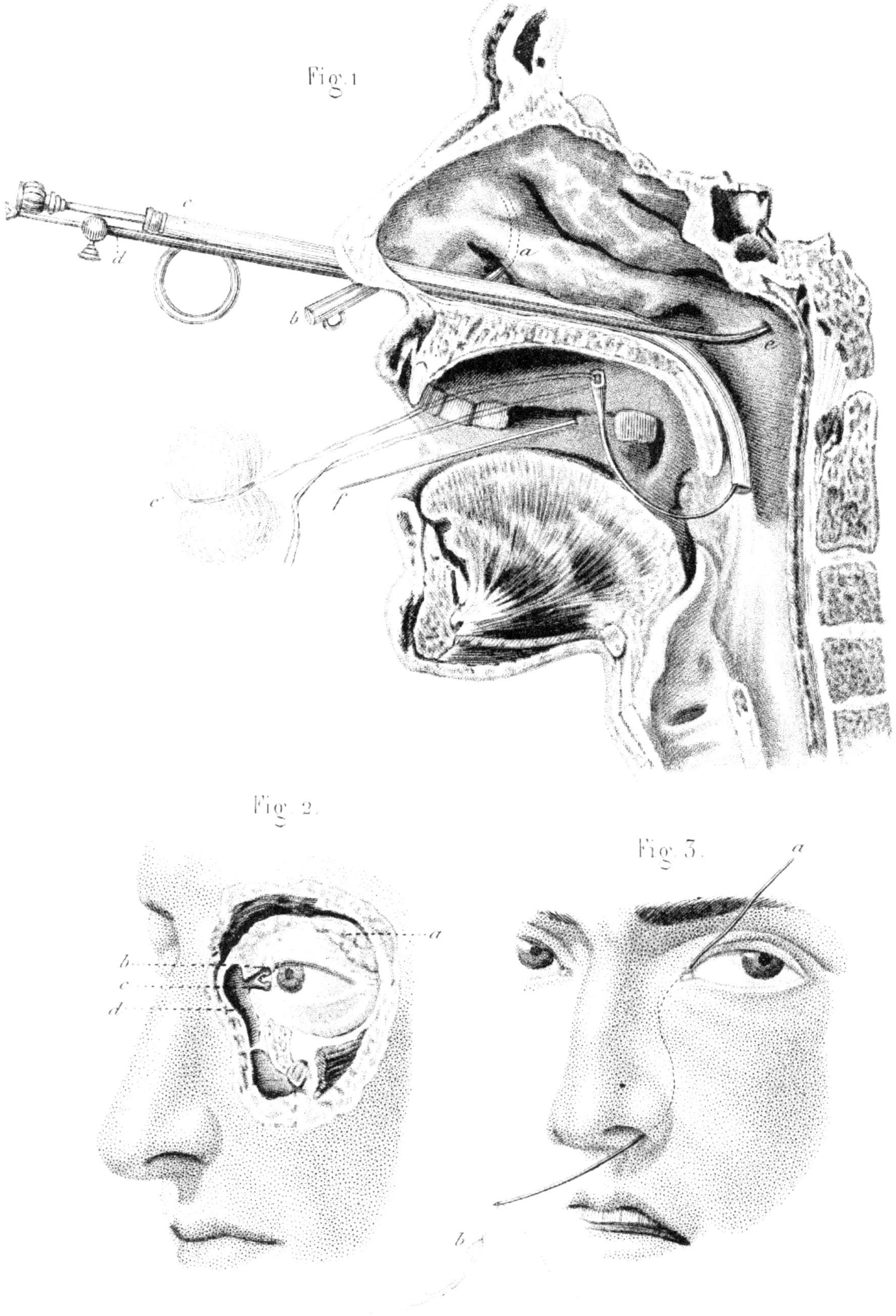

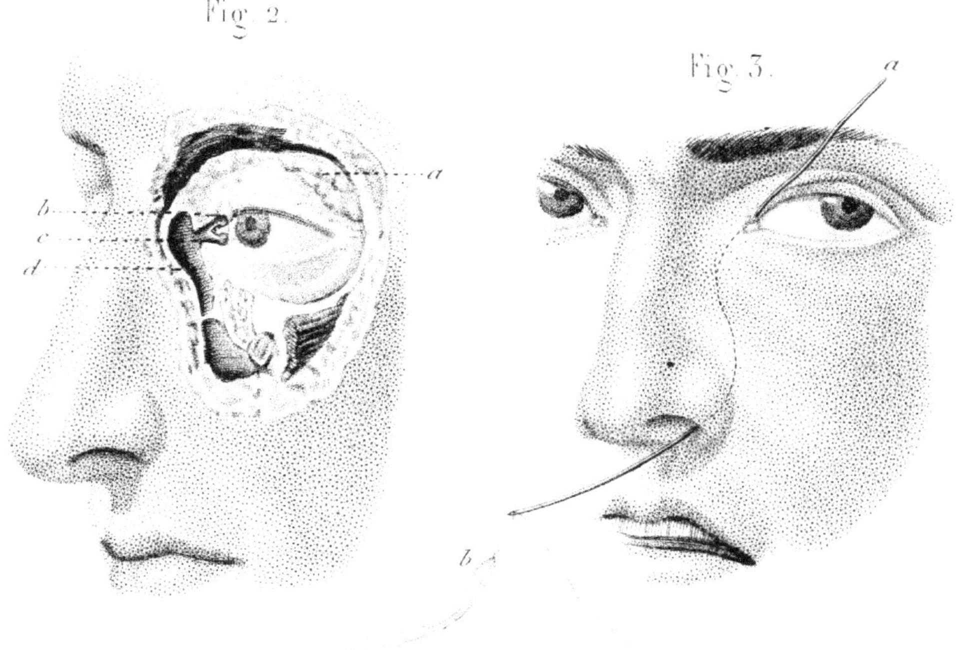




88: Diagram illustrating surgery on the lacrimal
gland.

89



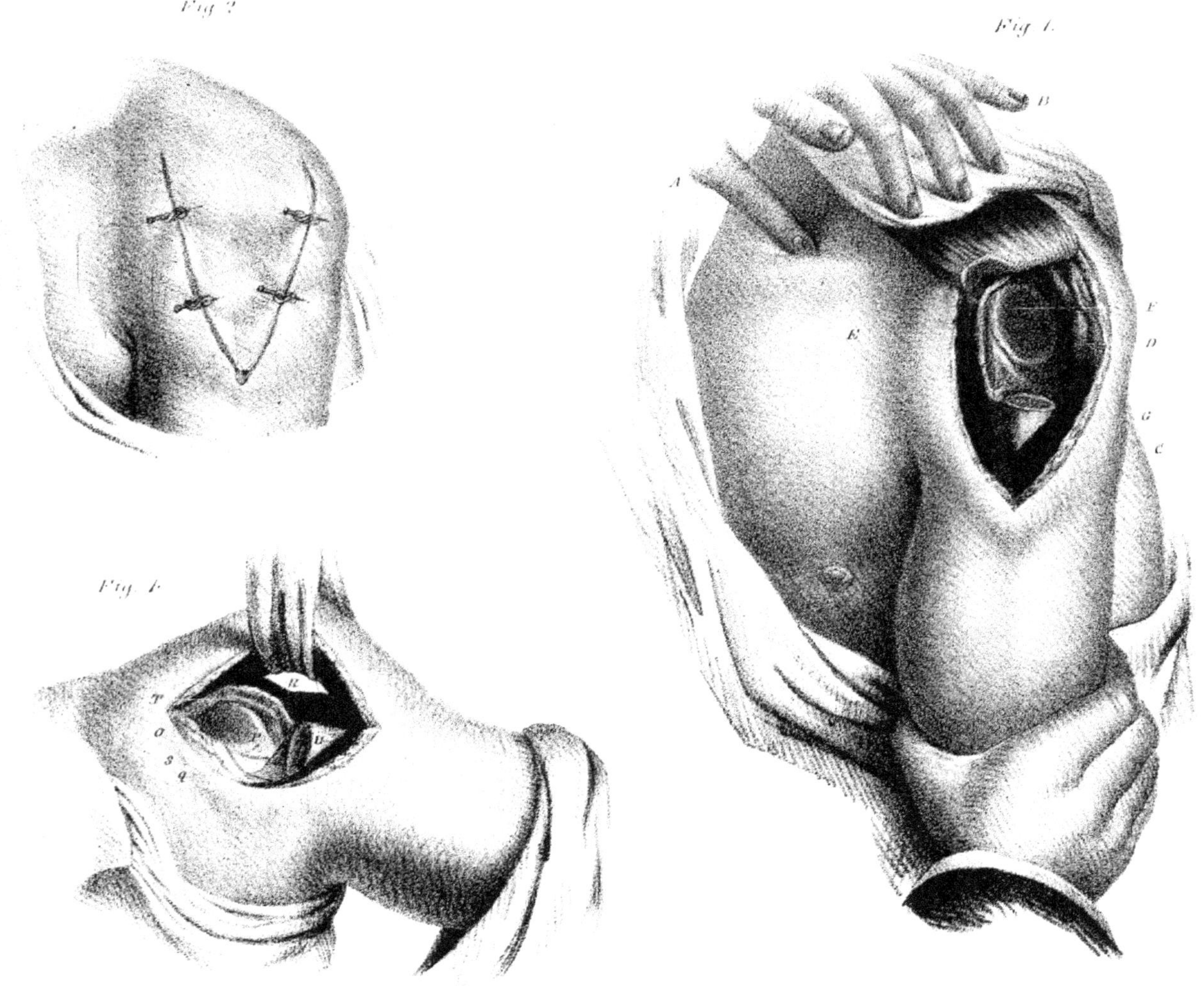


89: Diagram illustrating operative surgery of
the shoulder.

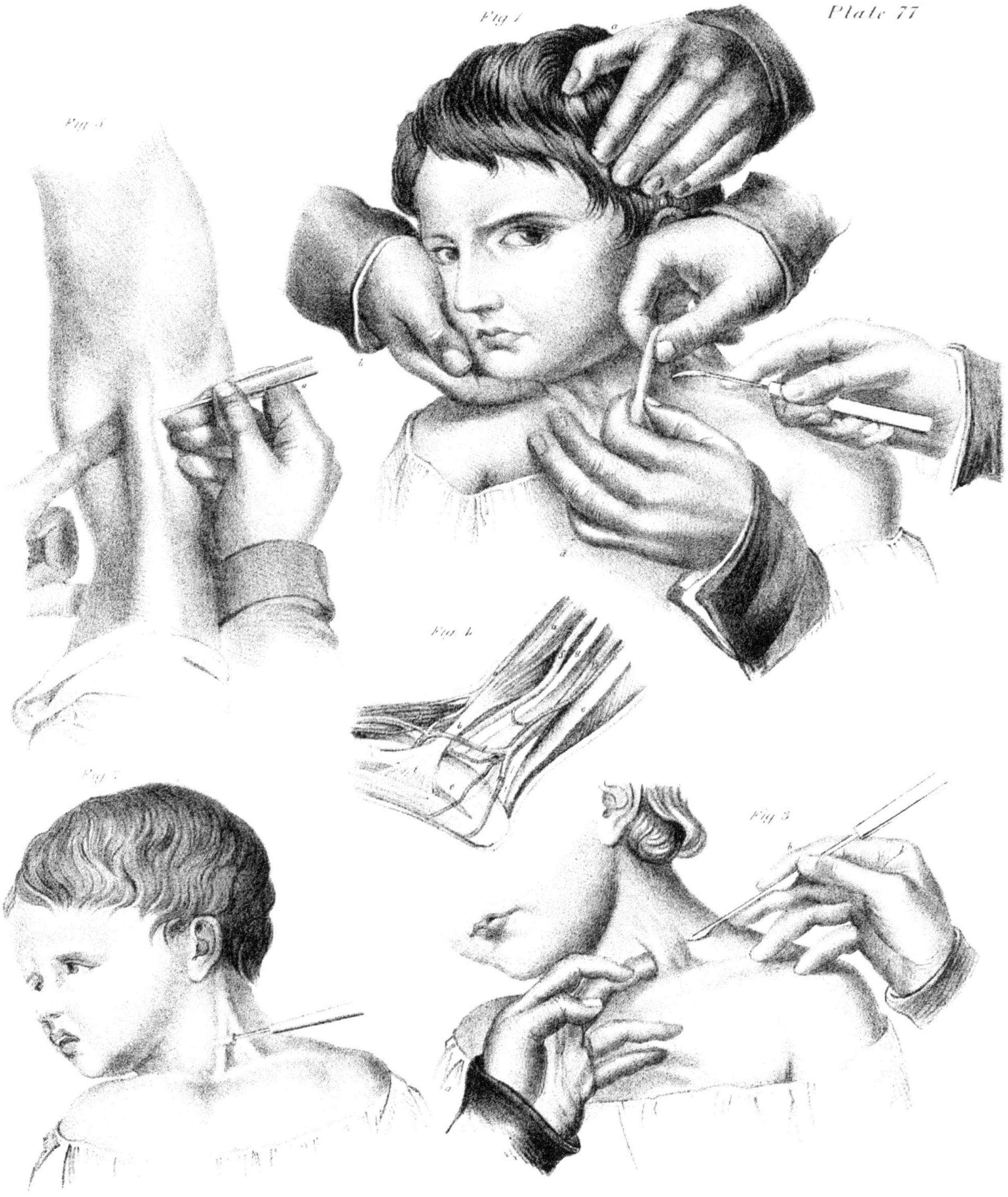

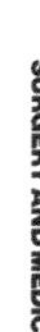


90: Diagram illustrating methods of operative
surgery to the neck.

91



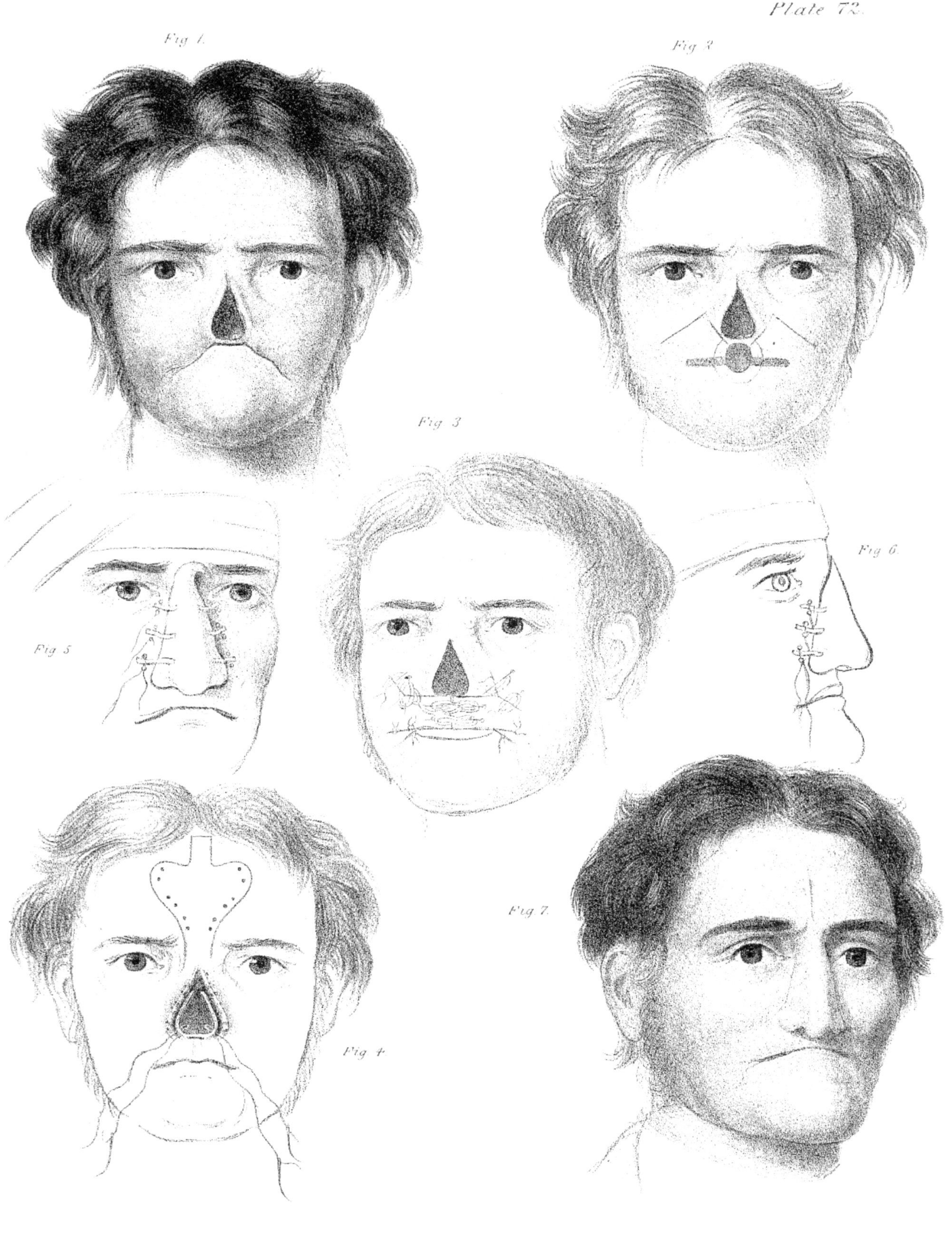


91: Diagram illustrating operative surgery of
the nose.

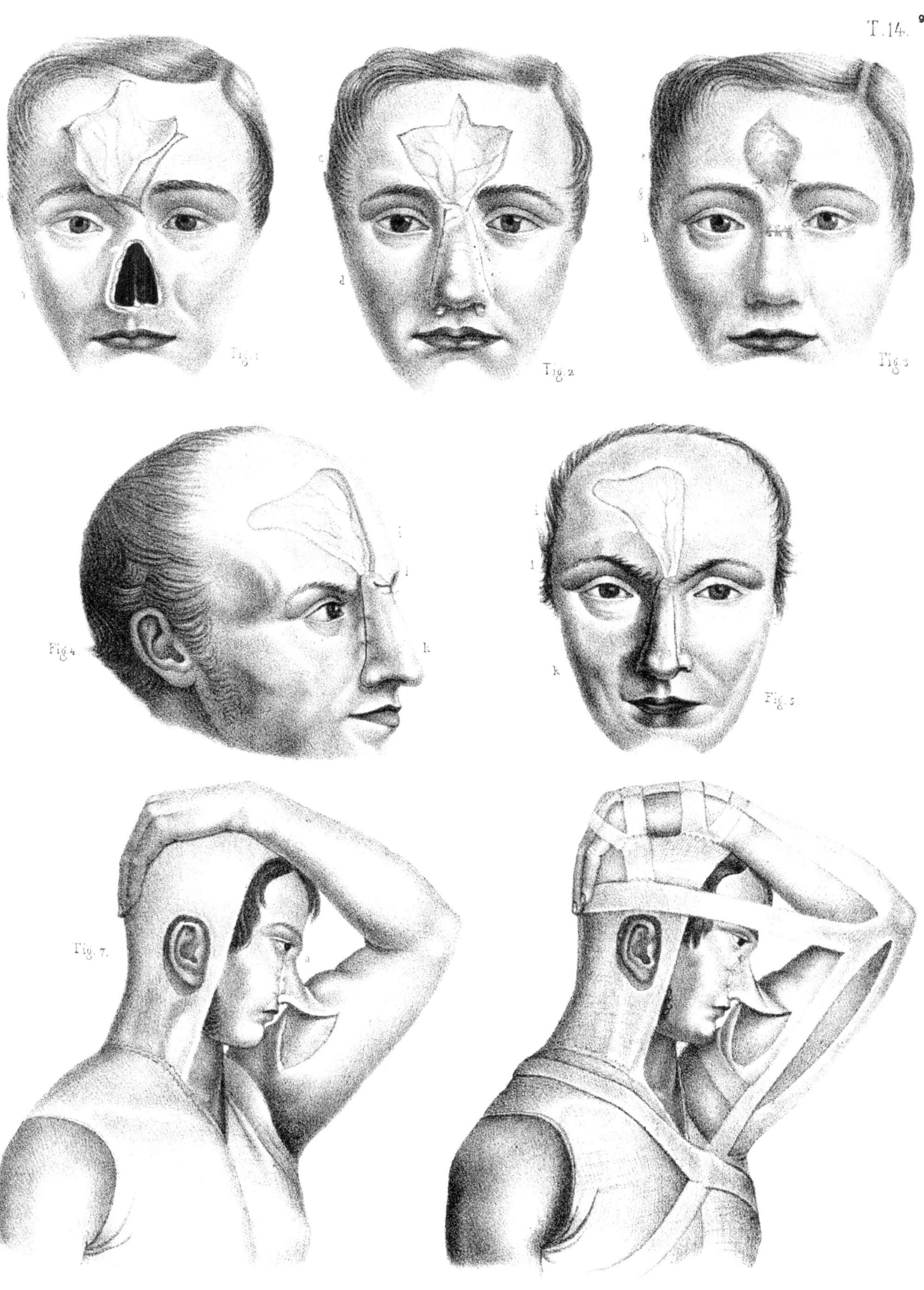




92: Diagram illustrating rhinoplasty.

93

*Plate 12.*



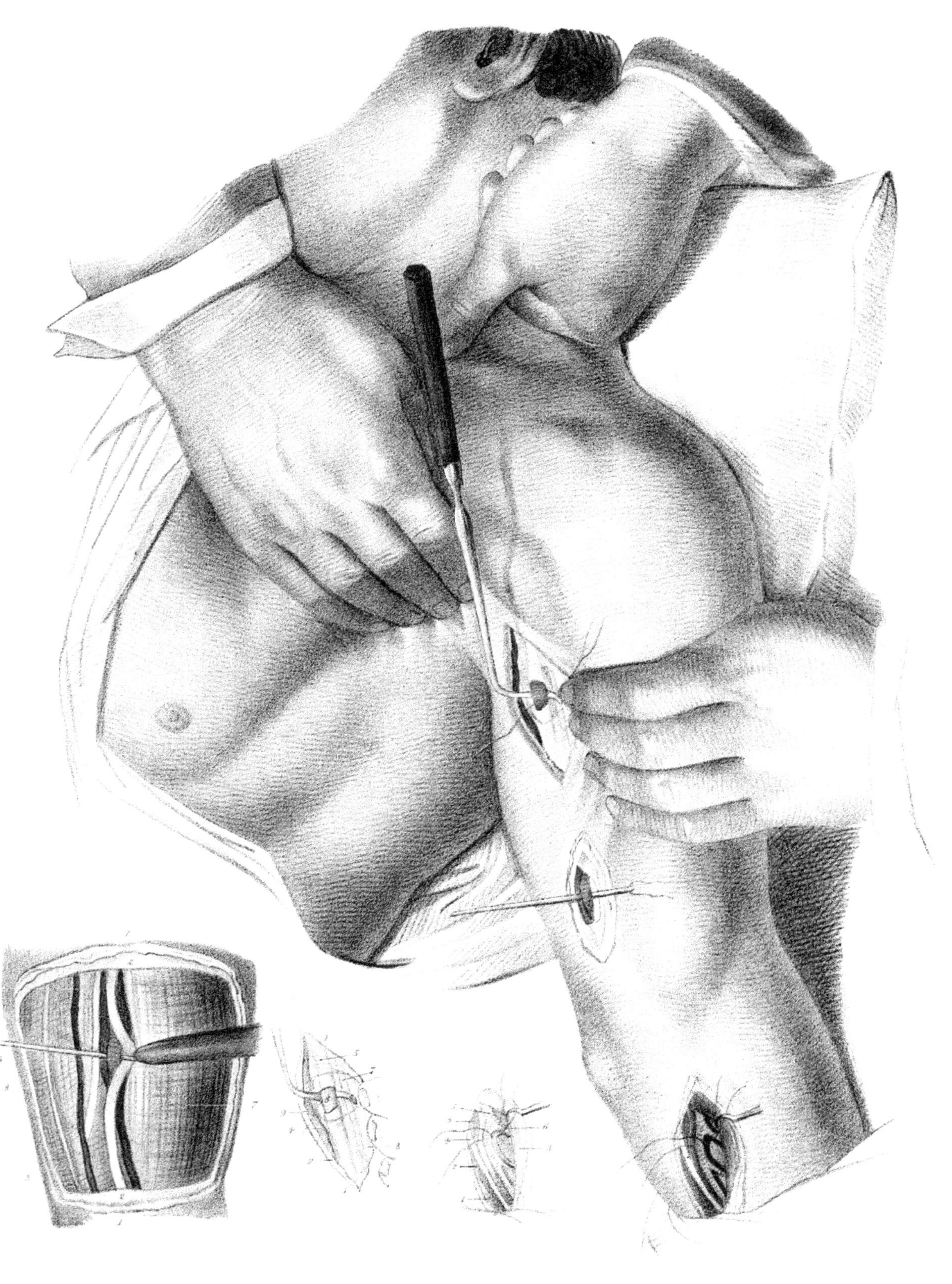

93: Diagram illustrating the ligature of the
humeral and ulnar arteries.

94

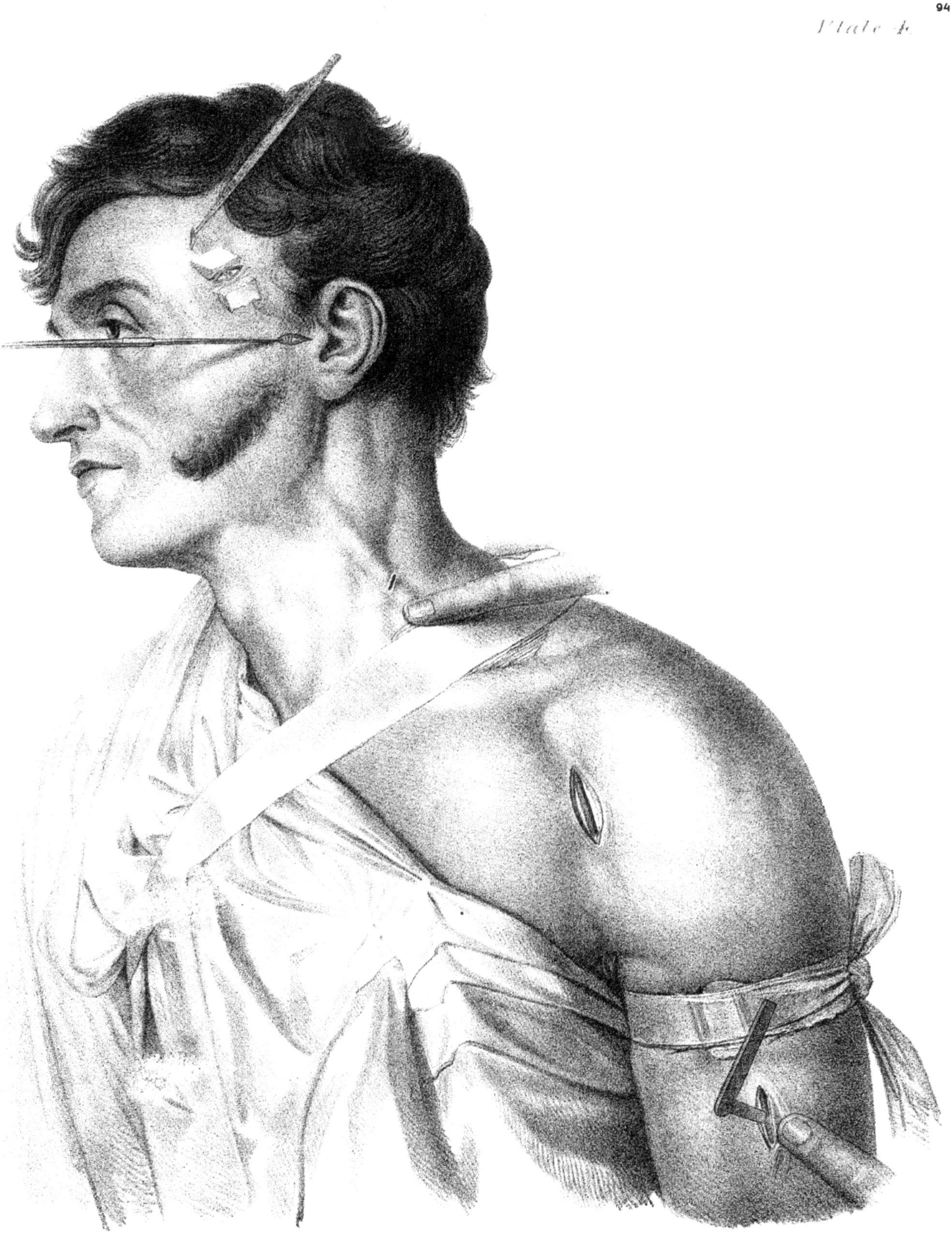

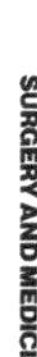



94: Diagram illustrating a treatise on operative
surgery.

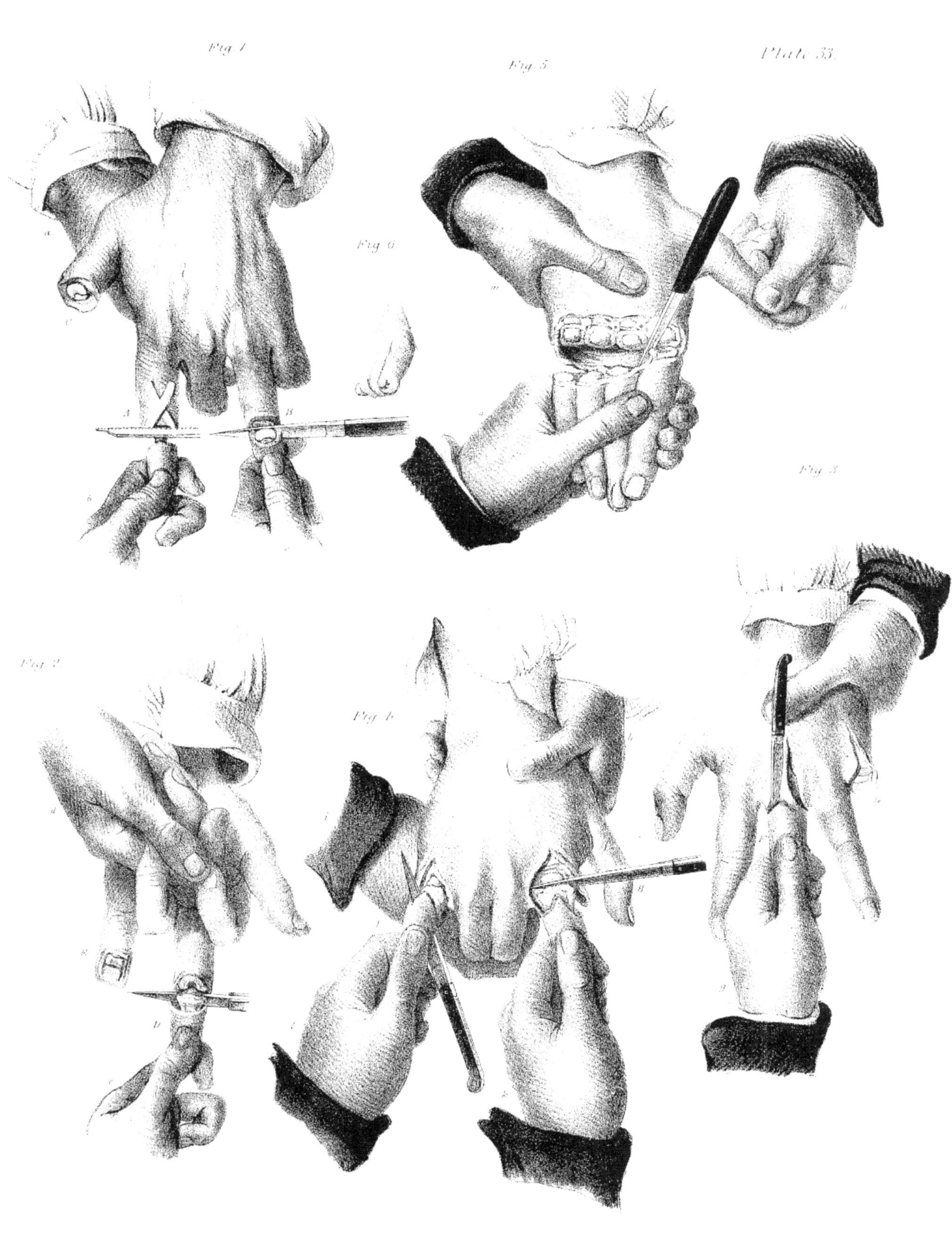


95: Diagram illustrating operative surgery of
the hand.

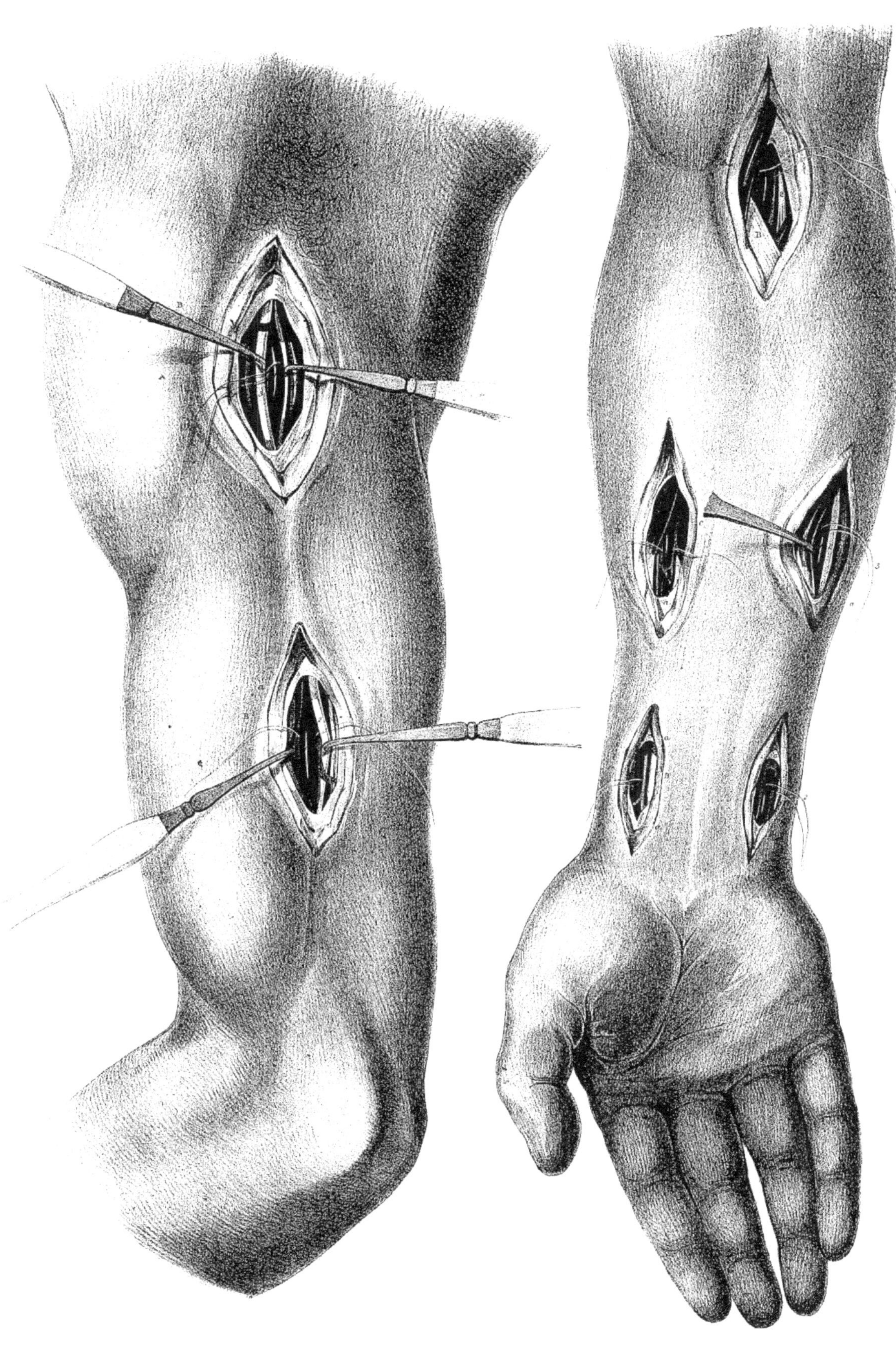

96: Diagram illustrating surgery on the arteries
of the arm.

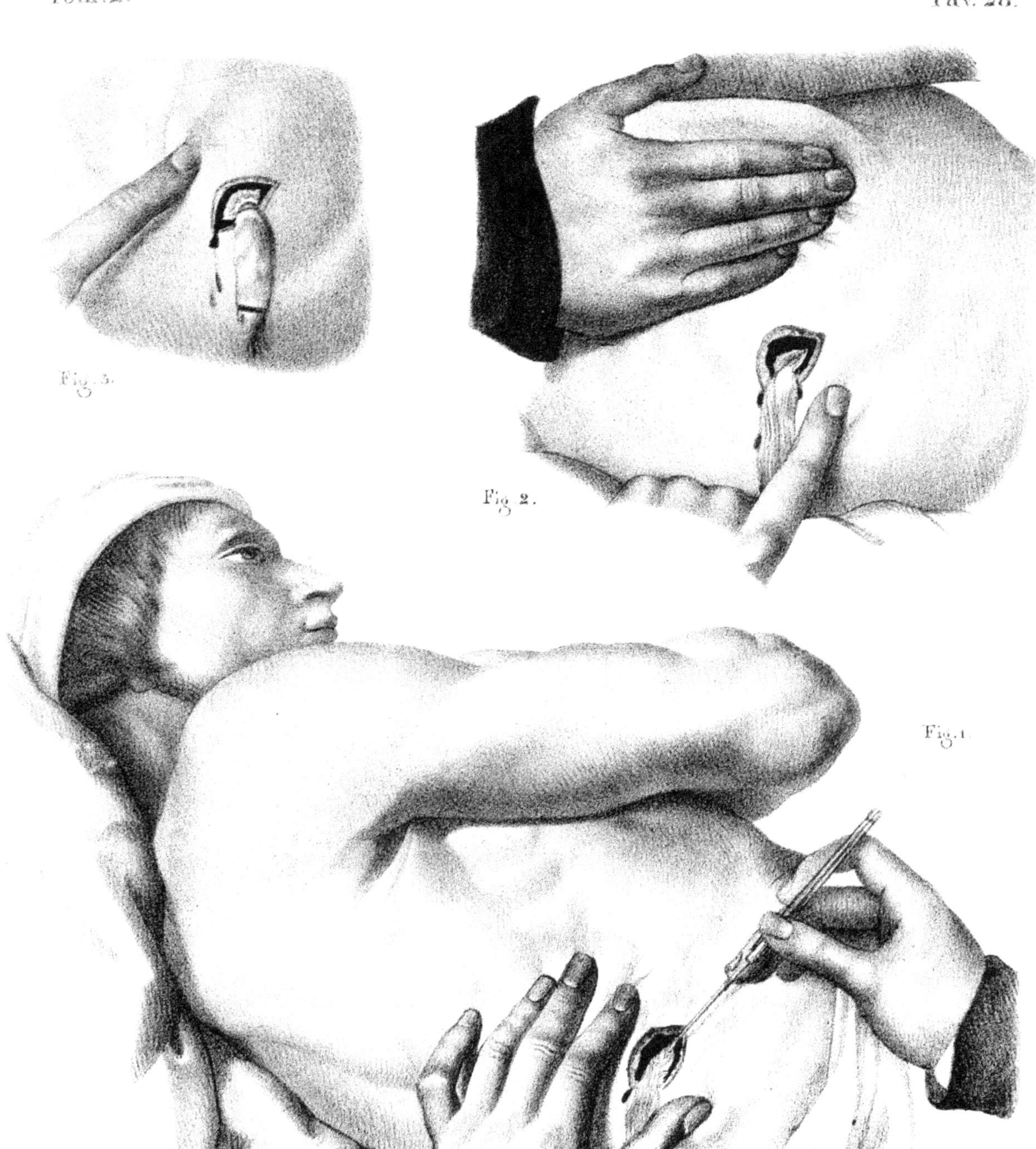


97: Diagram illustrating surgical drainage to
treat empyema.

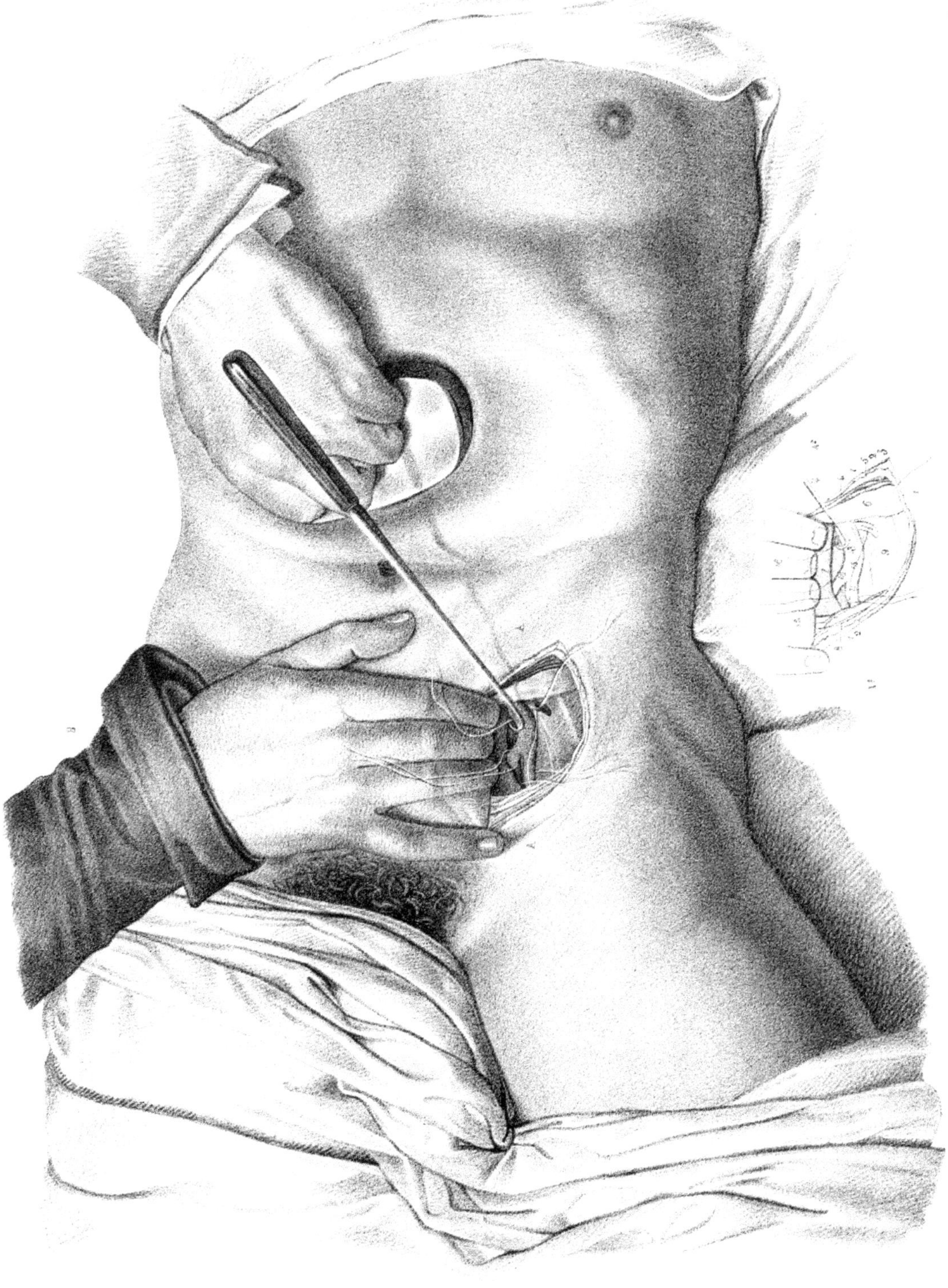

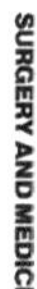

98: Diagram illustrating operative surgery.

99

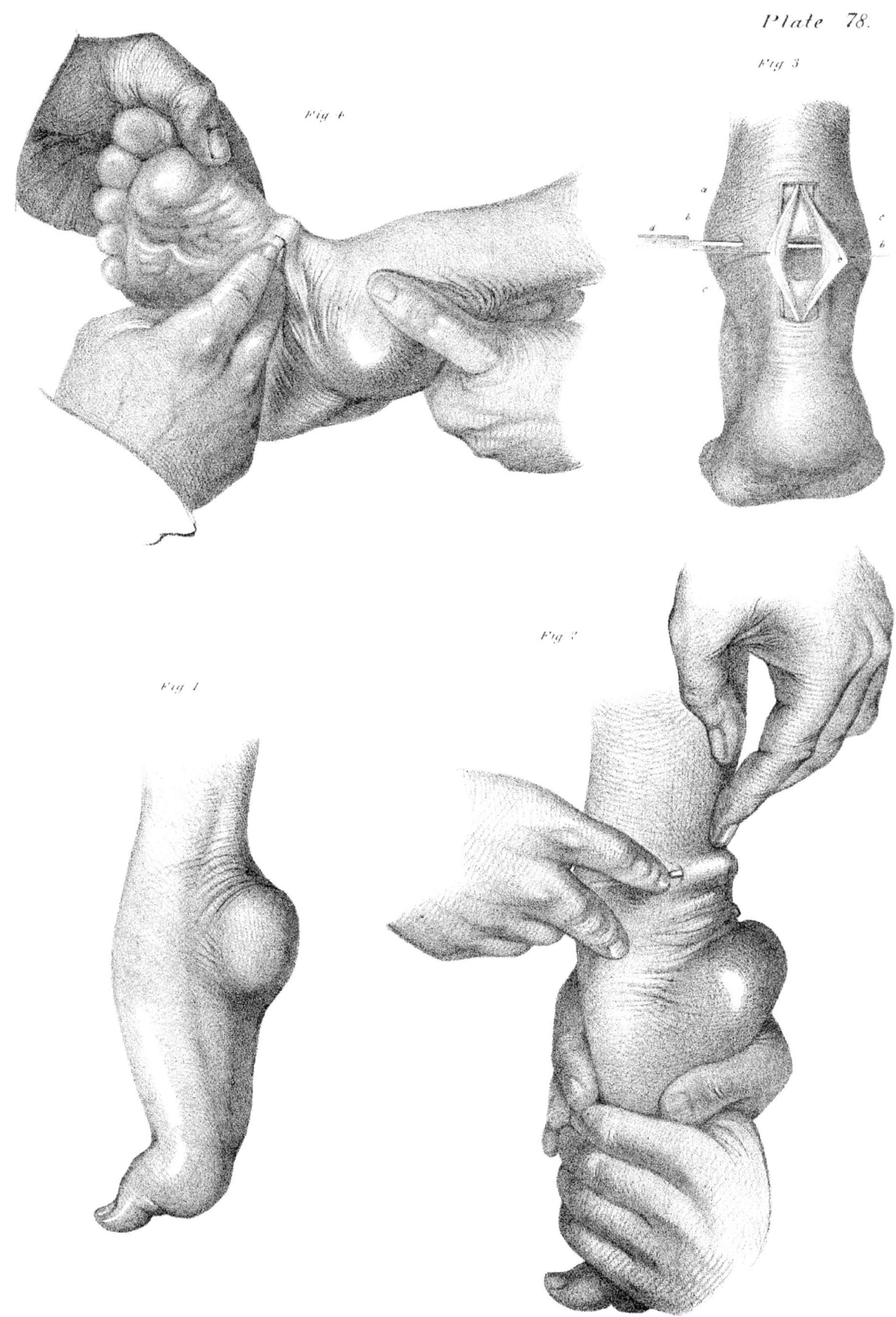


99: Diagram illustrating corrective surgical
techniques to repair club—foot.

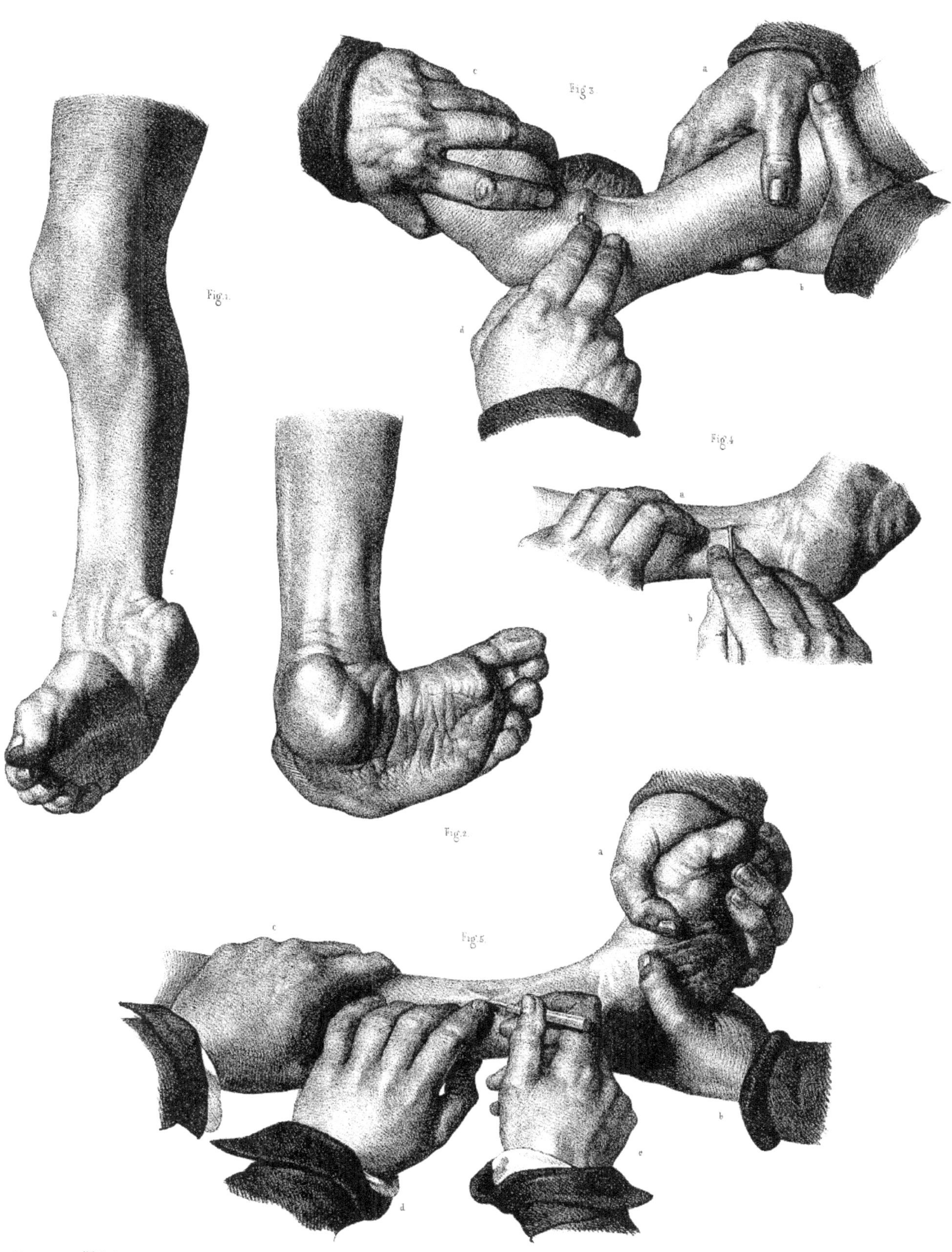




100: Diagram illustrating corrective surgical
techniques to repair club-foot.

101

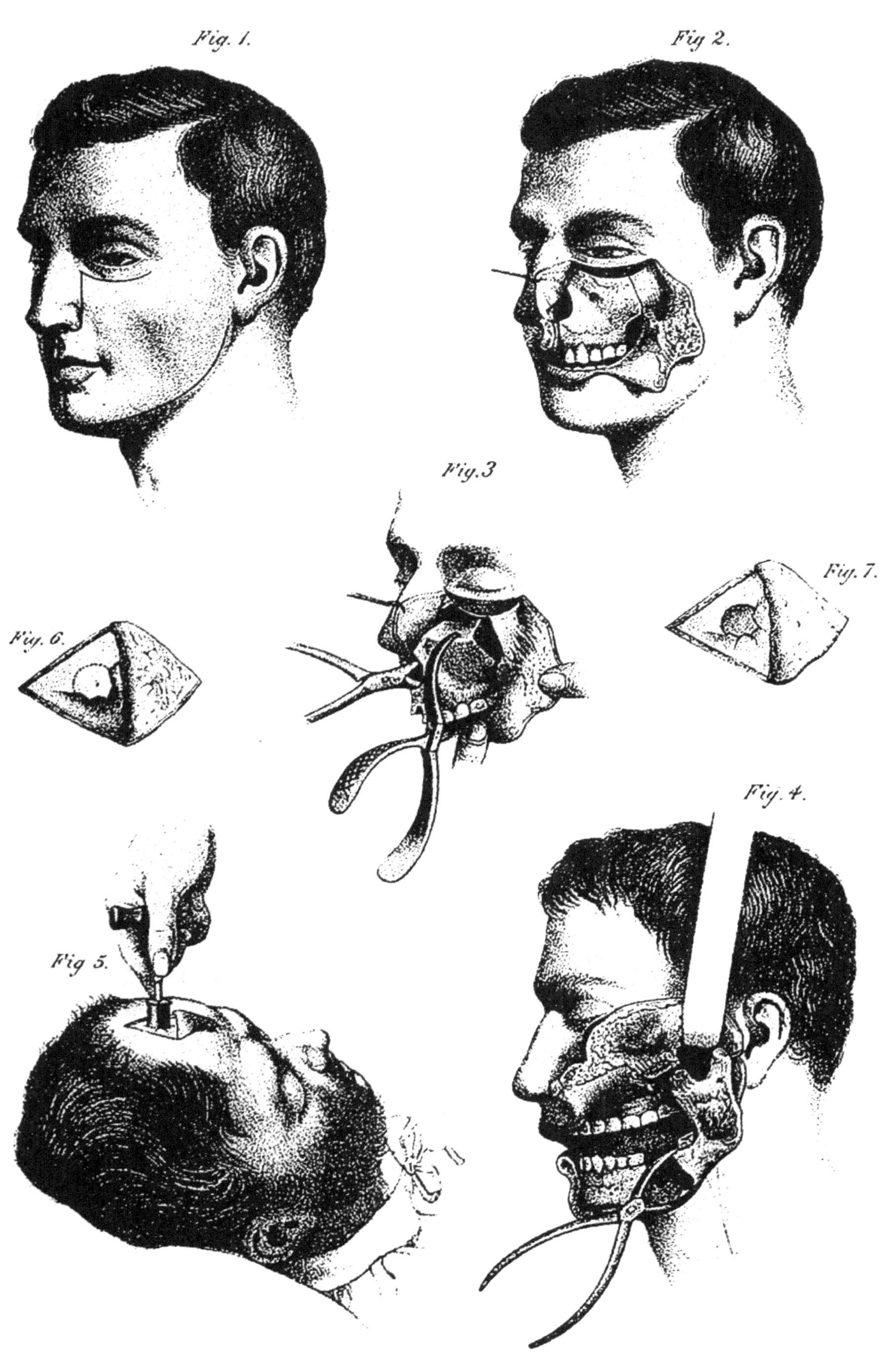




101: Diagram illustrating a cross—sections
through the human face and jaw.

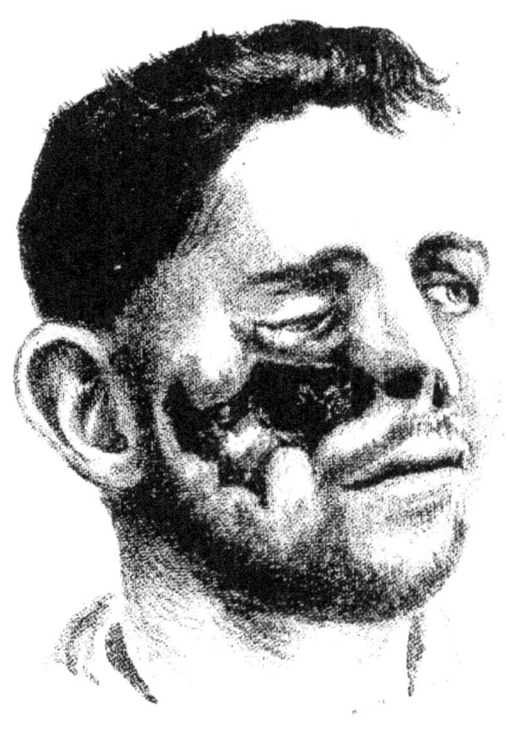
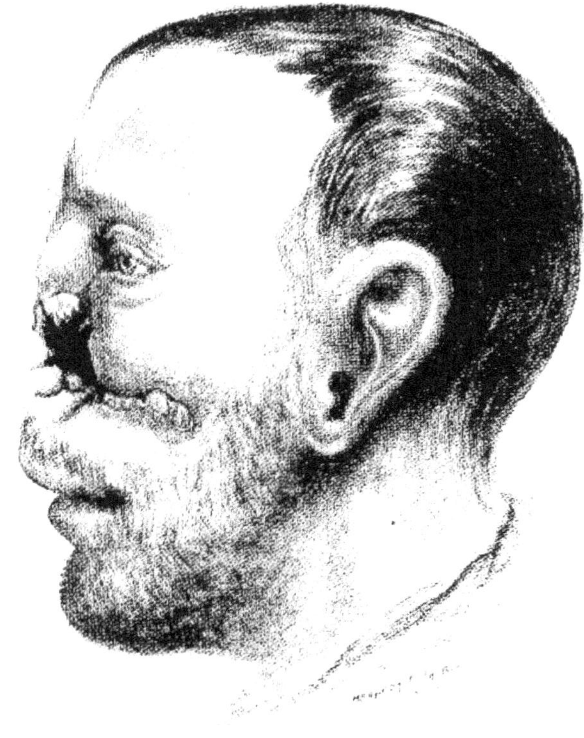
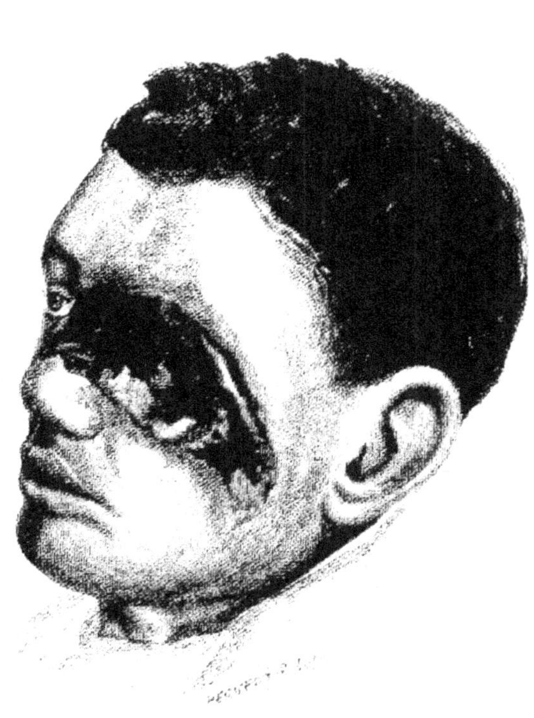
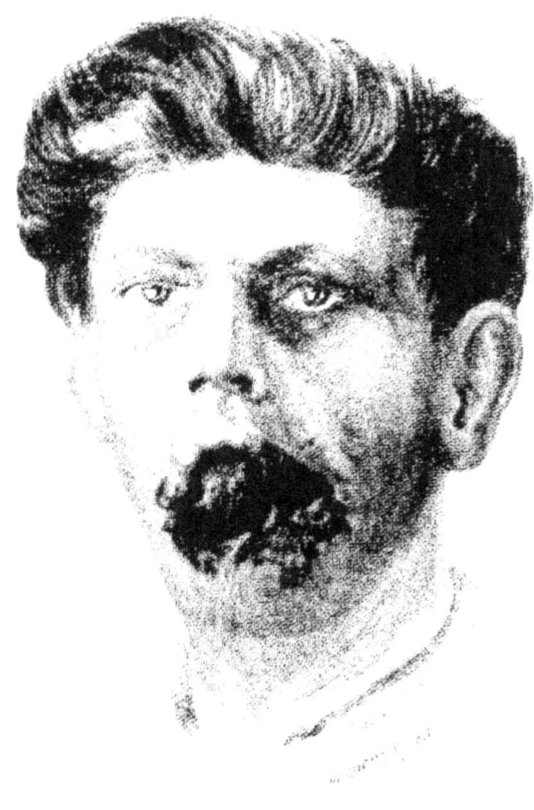



102: Diagram shows 4 male faces with injuries
sustained to the cheek, nose, eyes and mouth.

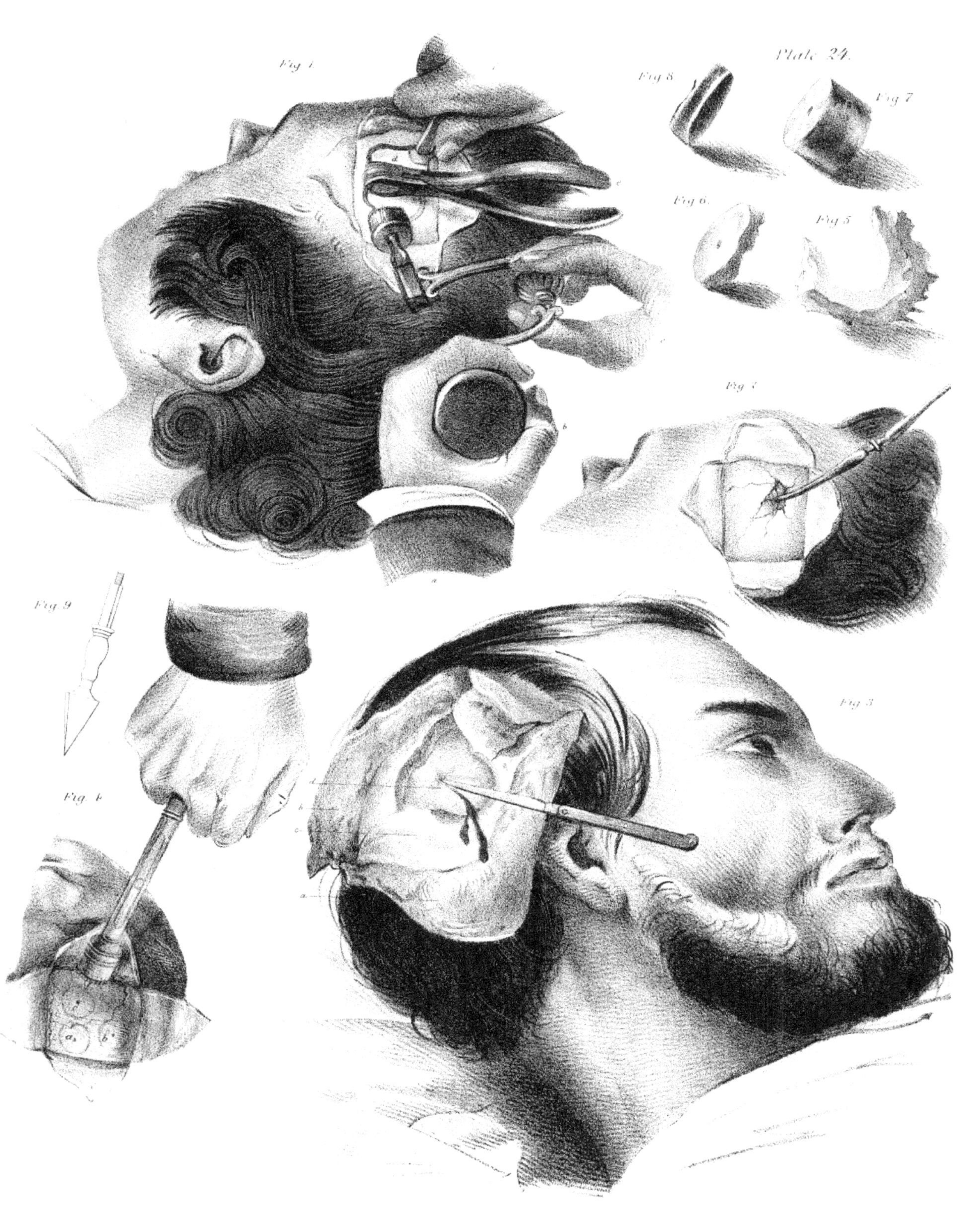


103: Diagram illustrates trepanation of the skull.

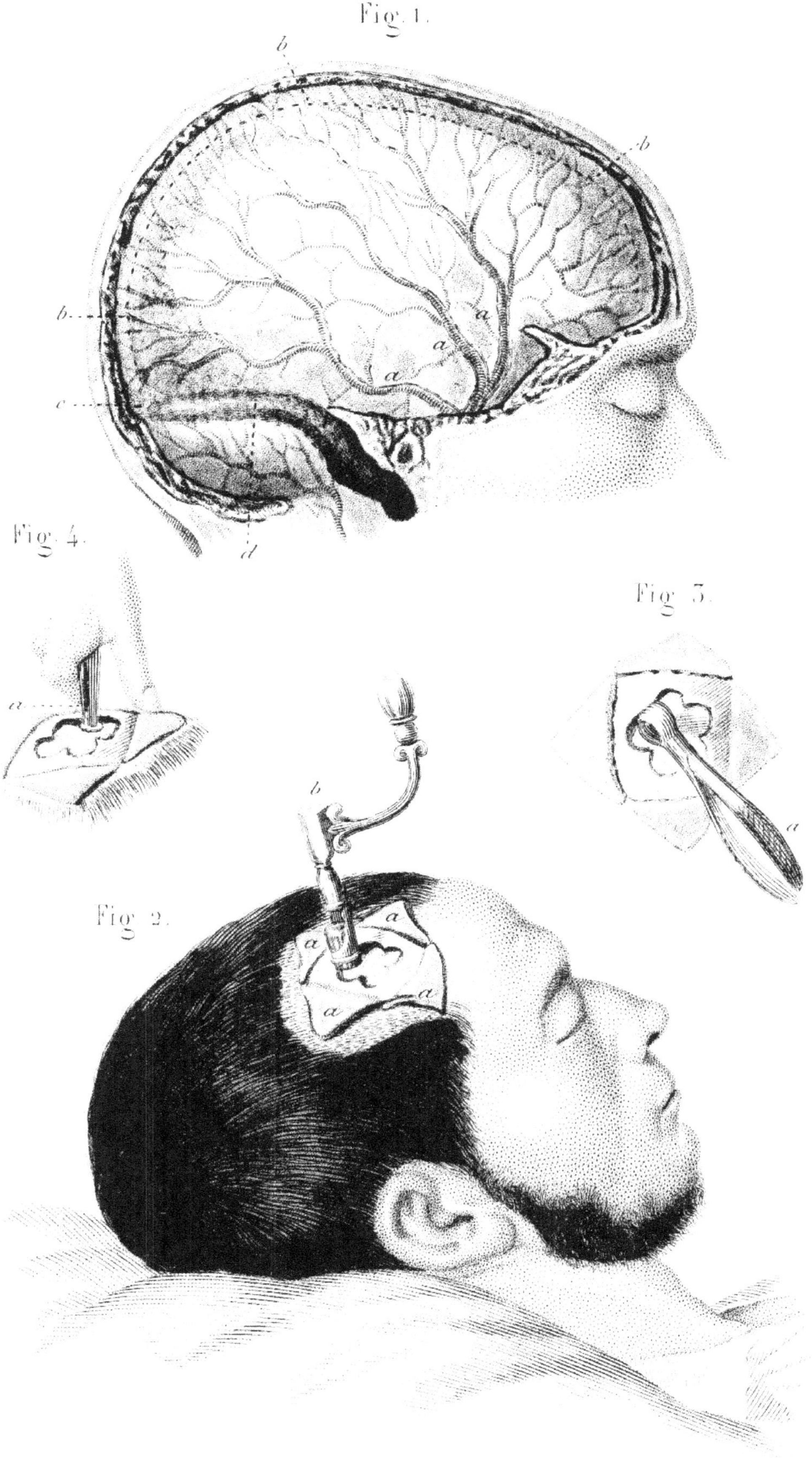


104: Diagram illustrates trepanation of the skull.

105

Fig. 1.

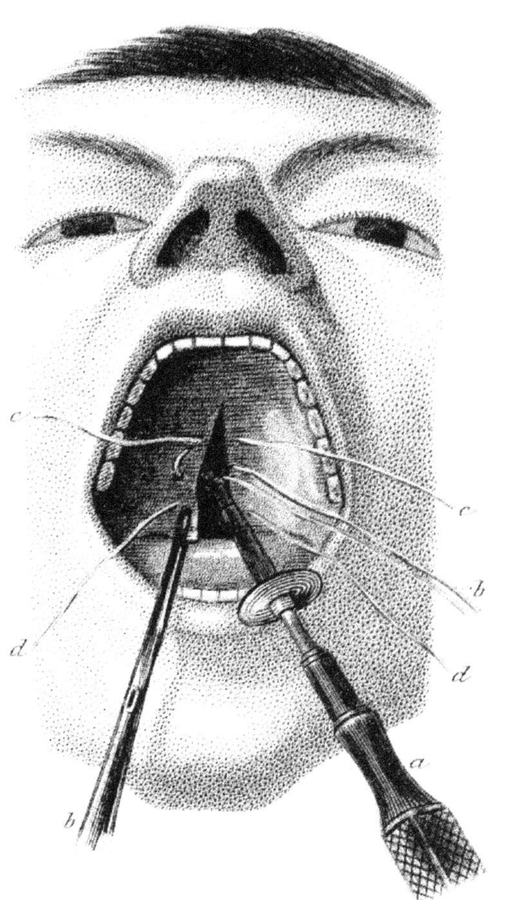


Fig. 2.

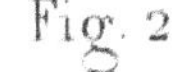
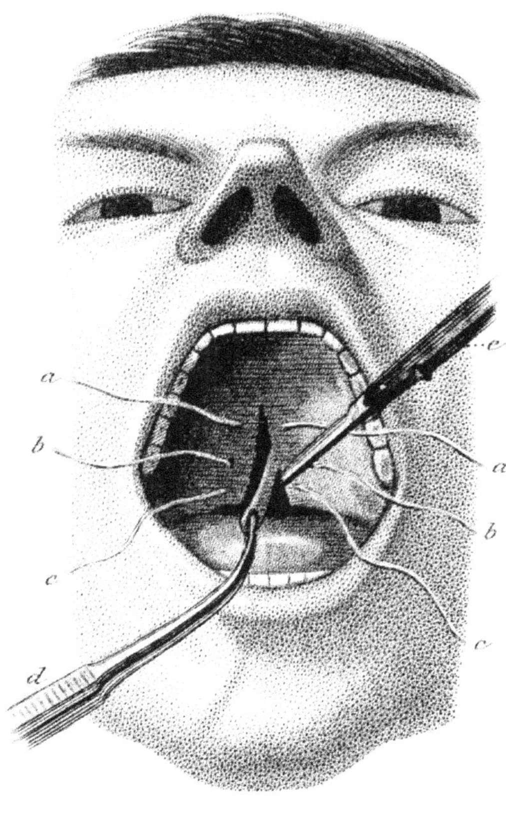


Fig. 3.

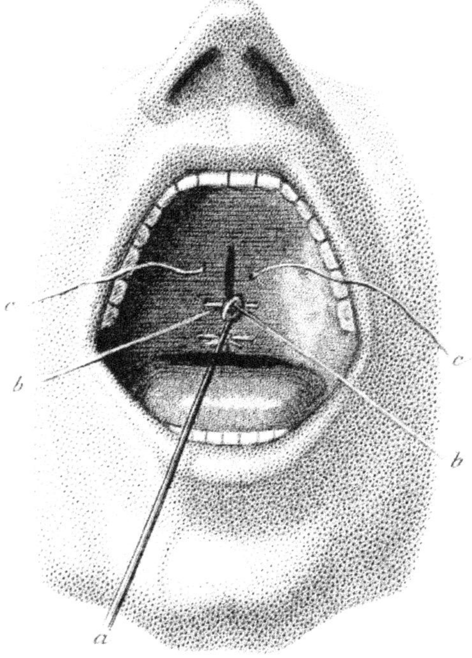


Fig. 4.

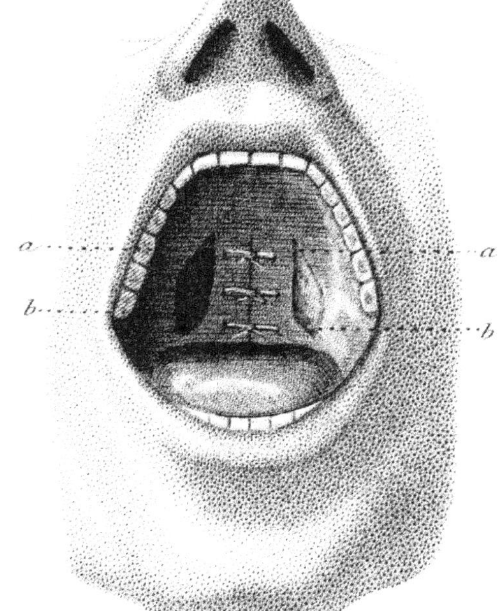




105: Diagram illustrates surgical repair of cleft palate.

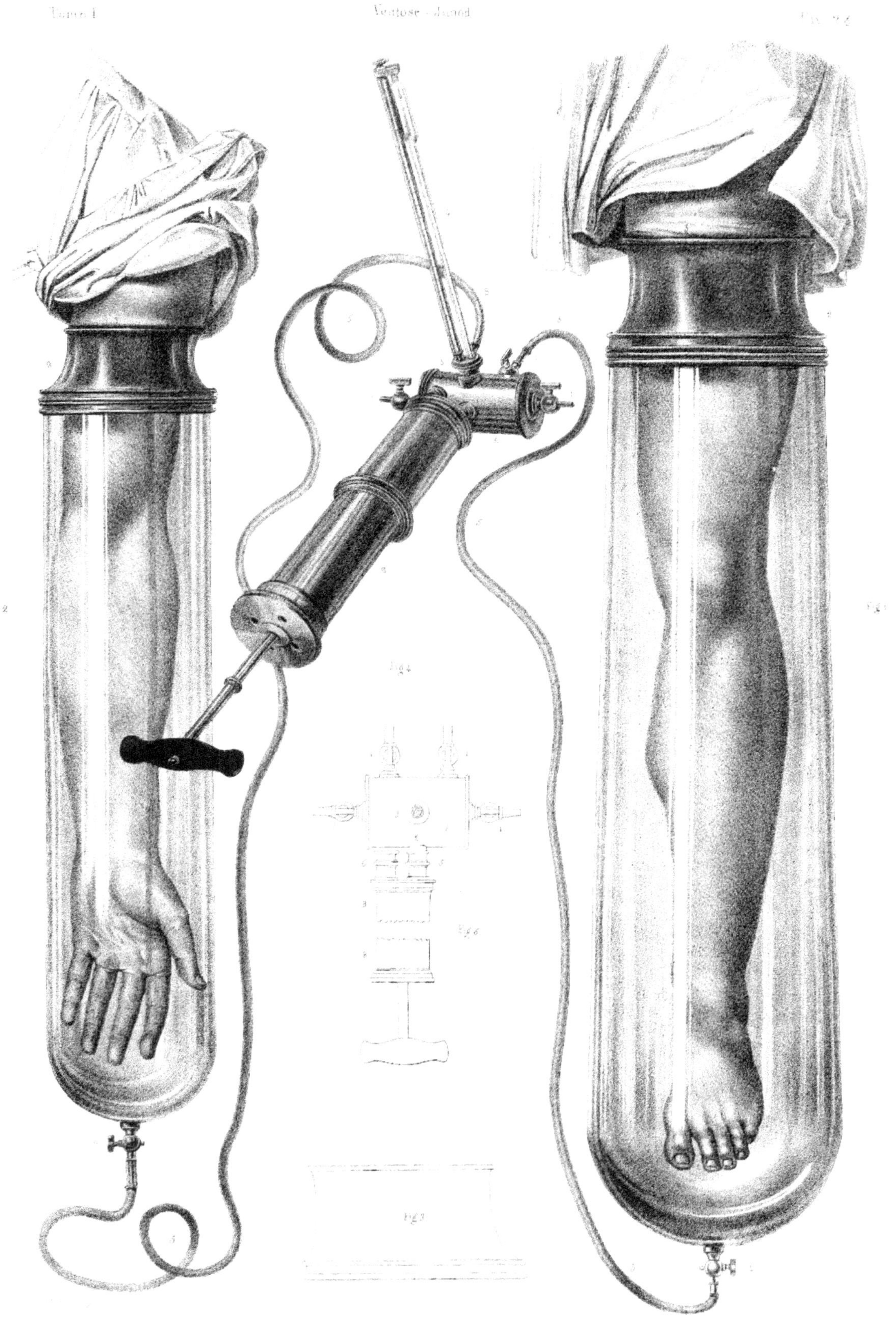

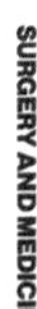



106: Diagram illustrates cupping devices for the
arm and leg.

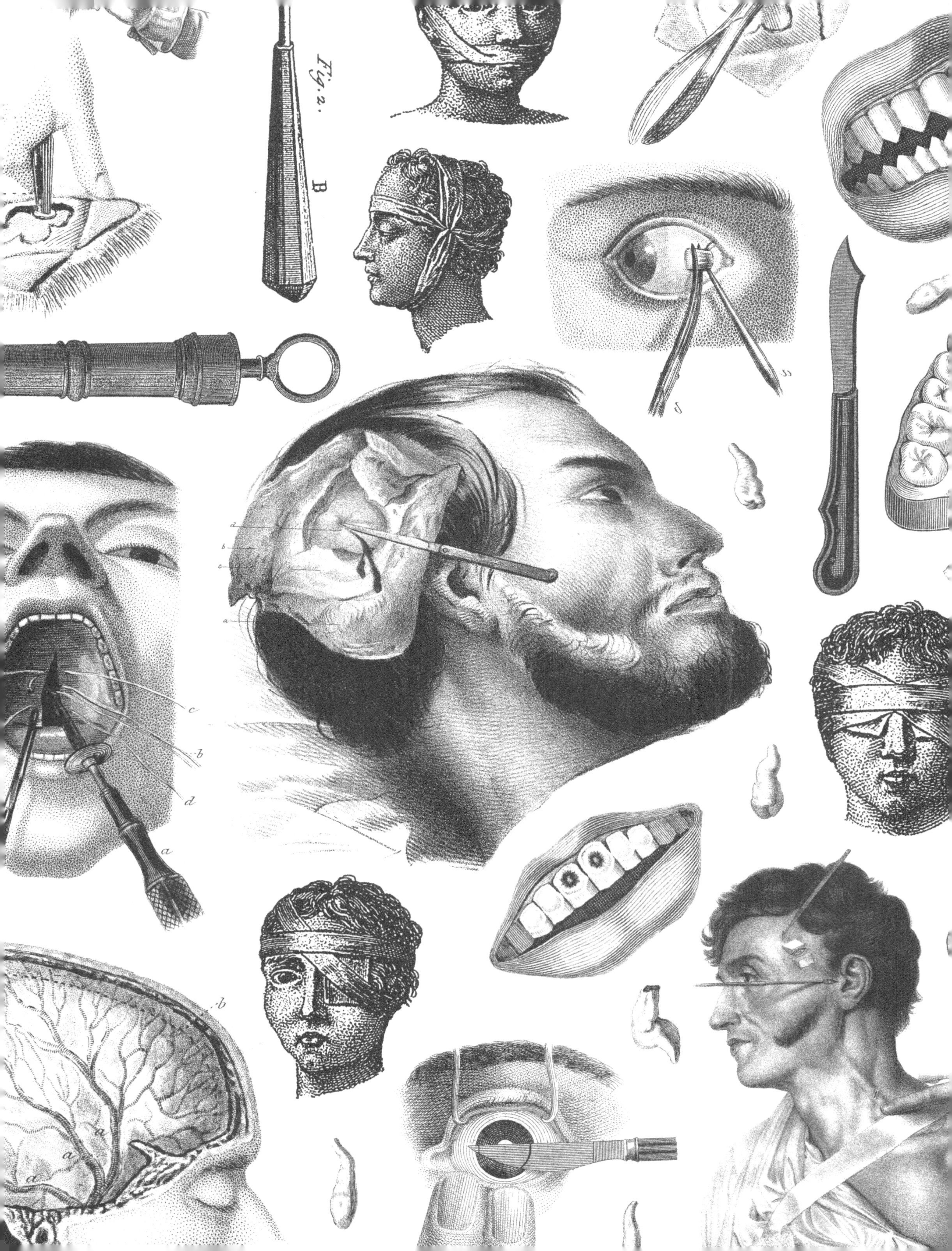

Fig.2.
B

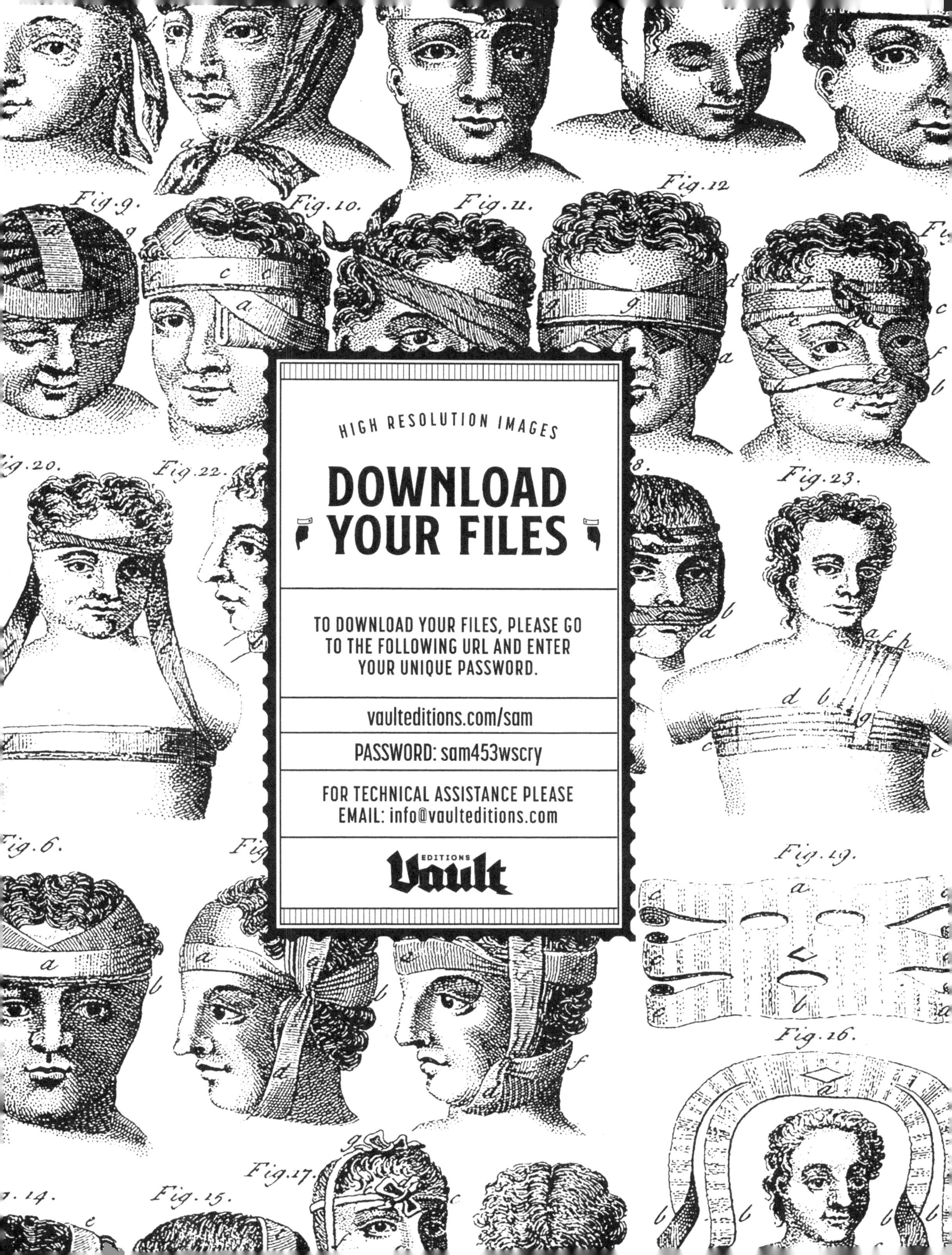

HIGH RESOLUTION IMAGES
DOWNLOAD YOUR FILES
TO DOWNLOAD YOUR FILES, PLEASE GO TO THE FOLLOWING URL AND ENTER YOUR UNIQUE PASSWORD.
vaulteditions.com/sam
PASSWORD: sam453wscry
FOR TECHNICAL ASSISTANCE PLEASE EMAIL: info@vaulteditions.com
EDITIONS
Vault